LET
FOOD
BE YOUR
MEDICINE

LET
FOOD
BE YOUR
MEDICINE

DIETARY CHANGES PROVEN TO
PREVENT OR REVERSE DISEASE

DON COLBERT, MD

WORTHY®
PUBLISHING

To my colleagues who, like me, continually strive to bring healing to those around us. It is our job to not only teach, treat, and comfort, but to also prevent the sicknesses that cause so much pain and suffering.

Picasso once said, "Only put off until tomorrow what you are willing to die having left undone."

I challenge all medical doctors to do more than just treat the symptoms. Find the root of the problem and treat that! Then you can put your head down on your pillow at night and rest assured that your patients are truly better off because you are their doctor.

CONTENTS

"The doctor of the future will give no medicine,
but will interest his patients in the care of the human frame,
in a proper diet, and in the cause and prevention of disease."

—

Thomas Edison (1847–1931),
light bulb inventor, with over a thousand patents
for inventions to his name

"Let food be thy medicine and medicine be thy food."

—

Hippocrates

FOREWORD

YOU COULD SAY that I've seen the results of this book firsthand. I would agree with you, but I would also say that I've lived it. It works, and it works well!

I watched Don as he battled through his own illness with amazing results. Begrudgingly, I will admit that I pleaded countless times with him to stop looking for answers that seemed "outside" the realms of approved medical practices, but I'm glad he persisted. What he has learned is life-changing.

We don't have time or space in this book to tell you all the stories of people whose lives were changed for the better because they simply followed the health regimen that Don recommended.

A few years ago, I watched as Don spoke to a crowd of more than 2,000 people. He listed most of the common diseases (i.e., arthritis, type 2 diabetes, heart disease, etc.) and then went on to explain how our bodies usually crave the very foods that fuel our diseases. He didn't focus on what they should not eat, but rather on what happens inside the body when the wrong foods are eaten.

Nobody left the room! They were spellbound. Don was fielding questions left and right until they finally called it a night. There was such hunger for health when people realized what was happening when they ate certain foods.

Now, for the first time, Don has placed this very information right out there for the world to see. It's right here. All you have to do is pick it up and apply it.

And what I love is that his teaching shows readers *why* and *how* and is not just a boring list of *dos* and *don'ts*. When you see the short-term and long-term benefits of taking action today, you are compelled to do just that! It will open your eyes.

But let me tell you where it begins. It starts with self-control, and you only get that by practicing it. You make good health choices each and every day. When you sit down to eat, ask yourself, *Am I choosing foods that bring life or foods that invite disease and death?*

I've had to do the same. We all do. The health you and I want is within our grasp. It will, however, take good choices to get there.

I can do it, and so can you.

—*Mary Colbert*

INTRODUCTION

YOU *CATCH* A COLD or the flu, but you *develop* heart disease, obesity, diabetes (type 2), dementia, hypertension, most cancers, and more health problems from the food choices you make.

That might sound like bad news, but the good news is trumpeting itself to the world: You can make good food choices that control, cure, or manage these very diseases. And not only are the diseases treatable, they are preventable as well!

On a practical level, it's a whole lot easier to prevent cancer, Alzheimer's, diabetes, heart attacks, and so forth than it is to treat them, but rest assured that we can do both.

That is what this book is all about—living a healthy lifestyle that both *treats* and *prevents* disease. And that is living life to its fullest. And *that* is incredibly exciting!

At the gut level, the reality level, people are people. They usually do whatever they want to do and don't change course until the last possible moment. It's human nature, especially when it comes to food and health.

Sadly, that "human nature" is driving full steam ahead off the cliff of ruined health, disease, death, financial loss, hurt, broken families, pain, and unfulfilled dreams.

However, people do *not* have to ride the train. They can get off any time they want. But maybe they've never heard that they are free to disembark. I don't know their reason for staying on board, but this I do know: the longer they wait, the tougher it will be.

My suggestion is to get off right now. Your health and your freedom await, and that is precisely what this book is about.

You *can* get off the train.

You *can* choose the life you want to live.

You *can* overcome.

You *can* beat your own genetics.

This is a lifestyle that brings life. It's not a diet or temporary fad. This is about health, healing, and prevention, and living to see another tomorrow.

WHAT AILS YOU?

If you are looking to cure, control, or manage a specific sickness, then 1) read Section One (chapters 1–5) as the basis of your thinking and planning and then feel free to 2) skip to the precise chapter in Section Two (chapters 6–12) that addresses your ailment.

I usually see the sickest of the sick on a daily basis. They need real answers for real diseases, and that is what I do. And the answers they so desperately need are more than prescribed medications. Treating the symptoms and not addressing the problem is an easy way to get frustrated.

Now, I'm not against medications for short-term needs. Thank goodness for medications, antibiotics, and more that save a lot of lives, for without them we might be dead. But you shouldn't start with medications every time. They can truly help, but they are usually not an answer or a cure.

The answers are found in the foods we eat and in addressing the core issue of inflammation in the body. Inflammation is the root cause of most chronic diseases, including cardiovascular disease, arthritis, Alzheimer's disease, Parkinson's disease, most cancers, autoimmune disease (such as rheumatoid arthritis, lupus, MS, colitis, Crohn's disease), and more.

Remove the thorn, metaphorically speaking, and the body heals. I don't have all the answers, but I have helped thousands of patients cure, manage, or control their sicknesses, and with great results!

If you, like me, want a healthy lifestyle that includes:

- healthy living now
- disease prevention
- weight loss
- treating the root of an issue, not the symptom
- a brighter future

. . . then keep reading!

—*Don Colbert, MD*

LET FOOD BE YOUR MEDICINE

SECTION ONE

Searching for Answers

CHAPTER ONE

℞

MY JOURNEY

Chapter One marks the beginning of Section One and the search for answers. It details my own journey, how I almost died and how I was forced to go on my own journey to healing. This is the same path that I take my patients on, only now it's faster and cheaper! This journey is the foundation to my belief that food can be my medicine and medicine can be my food!

Don Colbert, MD

DOWN BUT NOT OUT

IT WAS NO BIG DEAL. The year was 1983, I was in my third year of medical school, and I was fit as a fiddle. I had to run a three-mile race at my medical school as part of our fitness program.

The weather was not the best that day. It was in the high 90s with very high humidity. Not too unusual for Oklahoma summers, so the race went forward as scheduled.

If I finished the race with a good time, it would exempt me from running the race again until next year, and as a third-year medical student, I didn't have much free time. I figured I'd tail my avid-runner classmate, finish the race with a good speed, and be done with it. It was no big deal.

The race began and we went around the baseball stadium multiple times. On the last lap, about seventy-five yards from the finish line, something happened to my legs. I became extremely short of breath and my heart started to beat faster than I'd ever felt it. My legs suddenly were in excruciating pain, very weak, difficult to control, and I literally willed myself over the finish line.

Mary, my wife, was there at the race that day. She told me later, "It looked like your legs were broken or like you'd been hit by a car. You seemed to have no control over your legs."

When I crossed that finish line I collapsed to the ground,

foaming at the mouth, heart pounding, and gasping for air. The coach pulled me over to the sprinklers and hosed me off, but it didn't help. I didn't know it at the time, but my thigh muscles had experienced great trauma due to heat stroke. Quite literally, my thigh muscles burst! This released myoglobin (muscle proteins) into my bloodstream.

Across the street was the City of Faith hospital. They placed me in the back of a station wagon and drove me to the emergency entrance. All the doctors and nurses were outside looking at a massive storm that was approaching. They glanced at me as I was wheeled inside. I was soaking wet, but not from sweat. It looked like I was simply overheated, but the water was from the hosing my coach had given me. I was hot and dry on the inside. The nurse took my temperature and screamed for the doctor . . . I was 108 degrees and still cooking!

She knew, as I did (though I admit I wasn't thinking very clearly at the time), that body temperatures of 107 degrees or greater cause cell damage and internal organs can shut down. This can be deadly.

She screamed for the ER doctor. I stammered, "Put IVs in both arms."

They did, and the strangest thing happened. When those IV fluids started infusing in my veins, my skin pores opened and the perspiration squirted up like a miniature sprinkler system all over my body. Mary saw it as well. She said, "The water shot out one to two inches all over your body. It freaked me out."

Eventually, my mini-sprinklers closed down and my body began to absorb the IV liquids. The doctors figured I had simply overexerted myself and as a result had suffered heat exhaustion, and for that reason they sent me home. I wasn't home long before I had to go to the bathroom. My urine was the color of coffee!

At this point, I was very worried!

Back to the hospital we went and this time I was diagnosed with a heat stroke, massive rhabdomyolysis, and acute kidney failure. My ruptured thigh muscles released the muscle protein myoglobin, which was toxic to my kidneys, and all of it was trying to filter through my kidneys—thus the acute kidney failure. My CPK levels that monitored a muscle enzyme were the highest the hospital staff had ever seen.

As the muscles broke down my legs swelled, which caused extreme pain, and then the muscles shrank. All the while the healthcare staff kept me on a maximum flow of IV fluids so my kidneys wouldn't shut down, but my legs continued to shrink smaller and smaller. My once muscular thighs appeared smaller than my arms! As a male, that was both discouraging and embarrassing.

Appearance, however, wasn't the worst of the problem. The doctors didn't think I would ever walk again.

After doing a biopsy of my thigh muscles, where they took a sample of leg muscle from my skin layer all the way down to the bone, the report came back a few days later. Instead of telling me directly they talked to my wife, Mary, first. "He is never going to walk again," they explained. "His muscles are necrosed, or dead, completely . . . every layer, all the way to the bone."

She instructed them not to tell me right away because she knew I was in a delicate place emotionally and she felt that bad news would destroy my hope. Later she told me, "You are such a type-A personality, I could not see you living in a wheelchair all your life."

But the doctors told me anyway. Mary was livid and she told them, "You are all fired!"

"Mary," I argued, "You can't fire them; they are my professors."

That was true. Because I was in medical school, my doctors were also my teachers.

Mary and I argued and she stormed out of the room. In the elevator, on her way down, everything changed.

"I was not only angry at the doctors, I was reeling from the multiple blows," explains Mary. "From a no-big-deal race just a few days earlier to acute kidney failure to Don being wheelchair bound and then to possibly not finishing medical school, everything was spiraling down so quickly!"

Taking a deep breath, she began to pray. "That's when I heard the voice of the Lord speak so clearly to my heart," she says. "In my heart, I heard, 'He will run and not be weary; he will walk and not faint.'"

She pushed the elevator button back to my floor and came walking in with a resolute look on her face. She declared to me and everyone else in the room, "Man has said you wouldn't walk, but God has said you will."

That got my faith and hope back up. I knew somehow I would walk again and somehow I would finish medical school. I've always said faith and hope are critical as people walk through health issues. Now it was my turn to not only believe, but to also walk it out.

Eventually, I was released from the hospital. They sent me home in a wheelchair. My legs were dreadfully skinny. There was very little muscle on my bones. I couldn't even support my own weight and had to use my arms and wheelchair to get around.

As I meditated on the word of faith, I began to take a few steps and then a few more. It hurt severely but, bit by bit, I began to walk. Weeks later I walked back into that hospital. All the doctors and nurses clapped and were amazed. They had said I would never walk again, that the tissue was dead; but the muscles began to grow and to heal. I was, quite literally, a walking miracle.

After finishing medical school, we moved to central Florida, where I began my residency program in family practice, which was three years of working with other doctors before I could open my own private practice. Then in 1987, I started my solo practice in family medicine.

THE LAST STRAW

Running my own private practice meant that I was on call every single night, that I worked extremely hard, and that I had to start paying off my college debts. I had also bought a new car and a new home and opened a new office.

I loved practicing medicine. I had always wanted to be a doctor, to help people, and this was my chance. What's more, I was not wheelchair bound. I was walking and healthy. It was a dream come true. And though it was intense, I was loving it!

As I had studied nutrition and psychology while in medical school, it seemed natural for me to help my patients with their health, above and beyond prescribing medicines.

Losing weight was, and still is, a big need among many of my patients. I was doing a lot of diet counseling classes with patients. They would come in and I'd show them how to shop, how to cook, and how to go out to eat in restaurants (using the restaurants' own menus) and eat healthy. I would even take them to the grocery stores and show them healthy choices. It was the late 1980s and we were having tremendous success with the weight loss program.

Once a week, we had a group meeting. It was a great source of accountability and training. We were getting great results, and word spread rapidly through word of mouth.

One of my overweight patients, who had gone on the diet, was scheduled for arthroscopic knee surgery. I told her to go off the diet beforehand, but she chose not to. It was no big deal, as it was an easy outpatient-type surgery.

Three days following the knee surgery, while straining during a bowel movement, she suffered a massive stroke. She lived, and when she came out of the hospital, her husband sued the orthopedist, the hospital, the anesthesiologist . . . and me!

I didn't know much about lawsuits at the time, but she was suing me for $500,000, which was the limit of my malpractice insurance. I had only been in business for a year, which meant I had staff expenses, rent, setup costs, student loans, my own mortgage, and a car payment. I learned later the reason I was targeted was because I had a big insurance policy.

So we barreled ahead. Business was picking up speed, and that's what we needed. A local news reporter called and asked if she could film what I was doing with our weight loss program and interview me.

This was great news! All of central Florida would hear about us. More buzz and more awareness; it was perfect.

The reporter came to our regular weekly gathering of patients; some had lost twenty pounds, others had lost as many as seventy. They filmed as we discussed menus and talked about what foods we could order at restaurants. Then the reporter spoke up and said, while the cameras rolled, "Tell me about the patient who was on your diet and had a stroke."

The curtain lifted. It was then that I knew I had been set up!

It turned out that the attorney of the stroke patient was friends with the reporter. He probably figured the fastest way to get me to settle was to threaten to sabotage my business. They had no case against me, and he knew it, but that didn't stop him from lying and cheating.

The threat was out: They were going to "follow" my story—more like advertise my going-out-of-business story—if I didn't get my malpractice insurance company to pay up. Can you imagine trying to grow a business in a city where everyone thinks you almost killed one of your patients? That could really wipe out my new practice. It would totally cut the legs out from under me after being in practice for only one year.

I had been betrayed. I told Mary, "I'm going to lose everything." I didn't sleep for days. I fought depression on a daily basis. To say that I was stressed out would be putting it mildly! My prior heat-stroke had nearly destroyed my leg muscles and now the lawsuit was a major emotional blow to my psyche.

Oddly, my business actually grew throughout this time, but I felt it was all hanging by a thread.

I finally called a friend who was an attorney and told him to settle the case, and we did. I should have never done it, and would never do it today, but I wanted to be done with the matter before it destroyed everything. I knew that being the lead news story would be bad since I had been in practice only a few years!

It was heartbreaking, but the insurance company paid the un-just lawsuit and we moved forward. Mary was such a tremendous support, but we both felt the weight of the added financial burden to our already crazy, overworked lives.

I was free. With the legal issue behind us, I was ready to move on. What I didn't know was how far away my freedom really was!

UNEXPECTED RESULTS

It was a normal Florida morning, almost a year after the lawsuit, with the sun peeking over the pine trees. I had a lot of work to do at the office and that day would be another busy day.

I put one leg over the side of the bed and glanced down. My leg was fiery red! My arm was just as red. So was my other arm. I made a quick dash to the bathroom mirror. My body, except for my face, was covered with a red, itchy rash.

My first thought was that it was scabies. I had treated a patient the week before who had scabies. I put on the lotion to treat scabies, and then washed it off later as prescribed, but my condition only worsened. The itch was more intense and my skin was even redder!

For weeks, I tried every lotion I could get my hands on. Nothing worked. I started wearing long-sleeved shirts and rubber gloves so that I wouldn't scare my patients away. Who wants to be treated by an itchy, red, contagious-looking doctor?

> **REVELATION**
>
> I would do anything to get my health back! For most of us, we also need to reach that point.

Finally, after a month, I made an appointment with a friend who was a renowned dermatologist. I needed help!

In the exam room, he checked me out, then looked at me over the top of his glasses and stated matter-of-factly, "Sorry to inform you, Don, but you have the heartbreak of psoriasis."

I stammered, "But that's impossible. My heart has never been broken and there is nobody in my family with psoriasis."

His curt answer was, "I don't care what you say, you still have it."

There being no cure for psoriasis, much less a magic pill, he flipped open his pad and wrote me a prescription for coal tar. Coal tar is an orange ointment that smells like asphalt. Not a very patient-friendly treatment for a doctor to be wearing!

I smeared on the orange ointment and returned to work. "What's that smell?" my annoyed patients asked.

I itched and I scratched as I explained to my patients what that odor was, but my reassuring "Oh, it's not contagious" was not all that helpful. Long sleeves and gloves became my staple. It was miserable, and the orange ointment stained my clothes, my car, our sheets, and our towels . . . everything!

What's more, the skin would flake off, so much so that I felt like a snake shedding its skin. In my case, it was constant, from top to bottom, itching, scratching, and shedding. They say 70–90 percent of the dust in your home is made up of dead skin cells. I felt like I was solely responsible for that statistic.

The itch and rash were unbearable at times. I took no pictures, but if you ask Mary, she will be glad to tell you how bad I looked. They called me "Itchy and Scratchy" at home.

After six months of this insanity, I told my bathroom mirror, "There's got to be a better way . . . surely this isn't my future!"

I certainly hoped there was an answer . . . somewhere.

CHAPTER TWO

R̸

MY JOURNEY

Chapter Two is my "aha" moment, the time when my eyes were opened to the unexpected healing and damaging properties of food. It also details my passionate search for answers. When you are, as I was, ready to do anything to get healthy again, that is when things get interesting! The answers I finally found will both surprise and encourage you.

Don Colbert, MD

LET FOOD
BE YOUR MEDICINE

MY PSORIASIS RAGED ON, but I noticed that if I missed a few meals because I was busy, the itching was considerably better. Or if I drank just water or wheat grass for breakfast, I was amazed at how much less I itched. Even a dip in the ocean, the salt water, and sunlight seemed to decrease both the rash and the itching.

Conversely, when I had less sleep or was under extra stress, the rash and itching would get worse. I also noticed that when I ate certain foods, the rash would get much worse. After a big steak or bacon the next day the rash was far worse. I loved fried shrimp and would eat at those all-you-can-eat places, but the next day, I would feel like my entire body was on fire.

LOOKING FOR ANSWERS

A part of the Hippocratic Oath, which all medical doctors swear to uphold, states, "I will prevent disease whenever I can, for prevention is preferable to cure." The original Hippocratic Oath states, "With regard to healing the sick, I will devise and order for them the best diet, according to my judgment and means; and I will take care that they suffer no hurt or damage."

How could I have prevented my psoriasis? I asked myself that question hundreds of times. If there was an answer, I was going to find it.

It was also Hippocrates who said, "Let food be your medicine and medicine be your food."

If food should be my medicine and medicine should be my food, then perhaps what I ate or didn't eat could play a part in the treatment of my psoriasis. I wondered, but didn't have answers.

I admit, it took me a while to begin connecting the dots, but if diet, lifestyle, and nutrition played a part, I would figure it out. Scratching myself to death was not a pleasant choice. I simply had to find answers! The coal tar ointment would barely hold the itching in check, but it did nothing to cure the rash.

- I tried lotions and potions, and the results were minimal to nonexistent.
- I tried all types of supplements. Same poor results.
- I juiced, blended, and made smoothies out of everything. Still poor results.

It seemed that nothing could cure it. Nothing could take it away. But plenty of things would inflame it and make it worse.

As a medical doctor, I had been trained to address the symptoms, but after months and years of this, I really did feel as if I were going crazy. There had to be answers that addressed the root of the problem, not just the symptoms.

What was the root? Did the answer have to do with food?

It was in early 2000 that I tripped over an interstitial cystitis diet produced by the Interstitial Cystitis Association. Interstitial cystitis is also called "painful bladder syndrome" and with it you have bladder pressure and a painful "burning" sensation, ranging from mild to severe, when urinating.

I was intrigued because some people were being cured and the interstitial cystitis was being controlled. But what interested me the most was that their suggested treatment was focused on diet. In their brochure, ICA listed foods and beverages to avoid that triggered the painful symptoms. They had done enough research, no doubt by getting actual feedback from patients, to know which foods were most likely to increase the inflammation. Their recommended approach was to take it slow, to learn as you go, and to phase in and phase out certain foods that are safe or harmful for you.

One organ, the bladder, was really messed up by certain foods.

I began to wonder, "Could certain foods affect other parts of the body as well, like my skin?"

Triggers . . . food. Inflammation . . . one organ. One ailment . . . relief?

I knew that foods can be a trigger and cause inflammation, but to see that this same approach was being used to treat a specific ailment was very encouraging. If it worked

> ### REVELATION
>
> Treating the symptom is not the same as treating the root cause.

for that ailment, then maybe it would work for other inflammatory diseases!

If I could figure out what were my trigger foods and find out what caused my inflammation, could I also eventually cure my psoriasis? I hoped so, because I couldn't live like this anymore.

Sure, I may have struck out with two strikes, but the game of life was not over. I would get another chance to bat, and I was going to hit a home run! I was going to beat this thing . . . and I was not going to stop until I did.

The answer was food-related and I was going to find it, no matter the cost, no matter the time, and no matter the commitment.

LOOKING FOR ANSWERS . . . IN LEFT FIELD

This was the point at which my journey truly began. Searching for the answer to my psoriasis gave me an insatiable appetite for knowledge. I scoured the corners of the globe for every scrap of useful information that might help me. I attended seminars and studied under doctors who specialized in naturopathy, natural medicine, nutrition, chiropractic, acupuncture, biological dentistry, homeopathy, psychiatry, psychology, energy medicine, etc. You name it, I studied it.

I was out in "left field," as many would call it, talking to every expert I could get my hands on. I spent thousands of dollars traveling, taking classes, attending events, going to seminars and conferences, meeting people, and buying potions and lotions and pills.

I would run my medical practice on the weekdays and then spend almost every weekend traveling, studying, and learning. I was rabidly hungry, looking for my own cure. If it meant going outside my comfort zone, outside my area of expertise, outside my training, or outside my country, I was willing to do it.

Mary, however, was very worried about me during this answer-seeking phase. She writes rather candidly,

> To say that I was worried about Don is to put it mildly. I told him many times that he was going to lose his medical license if he kept up the insatiable rooting around for answers to his psoriasis problem.
>
> Talk about left field! I was sure that Don was becoming one of those "quacks" that we all hear about. I come

from a very traditional background, so I was beyond-the-shadow-of-doubt certain that my husband was going crazy. He would go to these strange meetings, talk to weird religious people, and interview countless natural "nuts."

Numerous times, I would call my friends and church members and tell them to be praying for Don. If I couldn't speak any sense into him, I hoped that God could!

Once, when we were at a small restaurant in a remote village in Hawaii, we happened to bump into an old, wizened doctor that Don had been reading about. I walked out of there, upset that Don would not let it rest and upset that he would waste his time with such crackpot people.

I was about to open my mouth and pray when God again spoke to my heart. This time, He said very sternly, "Get out of the way. Don't you think I love all my kids? Do you really think the American Medical Association is the only place where healing comes from? Don is going to bring healing to the nations."

That got my attention, and I shut up. I chose to do my best to support my husband, because I was persuaded he was going down the right path.

My medical training didn't give me the answers I was seeking. Much of what doctors learn after graduation is taught to them by pharmaceutical reps, so it is really hard to fault the doctors completely for this. They are bogged down and don't have the time, money, or resources to do what I did. I was motivated because I had a severe case of psoriasis, and it was a relentless taskmaster.

I don't fault the doctors, but I do fault the system. Doctors are so busy treating patients, doing paperwork, and figuring out how to bill for services, much less be paid, that we have come to rely on medical training from the pharmaceutical world. Admittedly, that's akin to the three little pigs asking the wolf for house-building tips.

At the surface level, in our grocery stores and in our refrigerators, our medical knowledge is here today and gone tomorrow. One minute you'll learn that margarine, potatoes, eggs, butter, low fat, protein, pork, you name it, is good for you, and the next minute you'll hear it's bad for you. I've said for decades that the mercury in fish was bad for our bodies, but I was called a quack for saying such a thing . . . yet now many doctors are saying the same thing.

> ## IMAGINE IF
>
> Doctors need to take continuing education classes every two years to stay licensed. Imagine if all medical doctors took just two classes on preventive health. That would transform things!

Practicing medicine really is that . . . practice!

Sadly, it's the same thing in the pharmaceutical world. While doctors don't get kickbacks for pharmaceutical sales, they may be liable when, a few years after recommending a new drug, it's discovered to have nasty side effects.

Mary adds,

Looking back, I realize how wrong I was to discourage Don from his pursuit of good health. A few years ago, we were with Dr. Oz on the *Dr. Oz* TV show, and he pointed to Don and said to the whole group, "This is the man. He is about to validate many of the things I've been telling you for years."

Thankfully, in this area, Don pressed forward in his search for answers and didn't listen to me.

My mind continually goes back to Hosea 4:6a, which plainly states, "My people are destroyed for lack of knowledge" (KJV). What about you? What about me? Do we lack knowledge in certain areas that, as a result, is negatively affecting us? No doubt that applies to every one of us!

In all honesty, when it came to the psoriasis that I used to suffer from, I would say that I was feeling pretty "destroyed" for lack of knowledge.

FINDING ANSWERS

Slowly, I began to put the pieces together. Looking backward from where I stood with psoriasis, I could see several milestones. What was it the dermatologist said to me? His exact words were that I had the "heartbreak of psoriasis."

It was true. I thought my baby of my medical practice was gone, destroyed in its first year by a frivolous lawsuit that was maliciously and manipulatively pushed through. And though I was not at fault, I was still embarrassed and ashamed. The guilt and betrayal made me angry just thinking about it! (It doesn't bother me now. It's part of my story, but back then it was a very raw subject.)

So I had indeed experienced a heartbreak, but who hasn't? Was my body so weak that I couldn't handle a bully and a financial loss?

Then I realized . . . my body *had* been weakened by the heatstroke those years before. My thigh muscles had burst and my kidneys nearly failed. Indeed, something had happened to my body that weakened it, and apparently that had set me up for the future.

Then along came the heartbreak and my body reacted, developing the autoimmune disease, psoriasis.

So if my body was weakened by the heatstroke and the trauma of the heartbreak lawsuit had driven me to the edge, then what was the trigger that pushed me over? The fact that I had gone over was not a question, for psoriasis was my very evident end result.

HEALTH

Trauma can flip a switch in our bodies that makes us susceptible to auto-immune diseases.

My mind was working overtime, trying to put the pieces together. Was there a specific food that was the trigger, the proverbial straw that broke the camel's back?

Talking to my mirror one morning, I asked myself, "Let's suppose it's a food that my body is now sensitive to—almost like an allergic reaction but not quite—then what food could it be?"

What's more, if a specific organ (like the bladder with the interstitial cystitis) could be affected by certain foods, then I was certain that my psoriasis was being affected by certain foods.

I took a food sensitivity test. It turned out I was highly sensitive to gluten and to peppers (red, green, jalapeno, and cayenne).

But I was eating these all the time! Every single day! I had gluten at every meal in the form of cereal or toast for breakfast, a turkey sandwich at lunch, and pasta or crackers or croutons at dinner. At the office, I would have chicken, rice, and beans with lots of salsa (which was loaded with peppers). I would pour the salsa on my rice and beans, dip my chicken in it, and then drink any salsa that remained. It's healthy, so why not!

How could these foods be hurting my body? They never affected me in any way before!

Obviously, the trauma of my heatstroke had damaged my body, and then the emotional trauma, which was the heartbreak of the lawsuit, had flipped a switch inside of me, triggering the autoimmune disease psoriasis. I also knew that food sensitivity meant inflammation. When you are sensitive to something, it's usually inflaming you on the inside.

Since it was gluten and peppers causing my inflammation, I surmised that my small intestine (where the food is absorbed into your body) was paying a price for it.

I then had lab tests performed that showed my small intestine had increased intestinal permeability. This meant that microscopic holes had developed in the intestine wall, which essentially allowed the proteins and peptides from the food I ate to leak (at the microscopic level) directly into my body.

My small intestine was inflamed and a mess, but I knew that the skin was a natural reflection of the small intestine. I was inflamed on the inside, and my skin was inflamed on the outside. The gluten and peppers were my thorns that had inflamed my small intestines.

> **FACTOID**
>
> We forget 98% of what we have heard within one month. Feel free to use a highlighter and mark up this book!

At that point, the answer was obvious: get off gluten and peppers as quickly as possible!

Would it cure me? I didn't know, but at least I knew my next step. And getting my intestines healthy again would certainly be a key move.

I immediately quit eating gluten and peppers. It wasn't easy, but if it would bring some relief, I was going to do it. Knowing that my intestine was out of balance, I also took probiotics, some supplements to kill yeast and parasites, oregano to kill the bad bacteria, and some nutrients to repair my small intestine. (See "Appendix D: Alcat Testing" to find out how you can discover what foods your body reacts to and why.)

Within three to four months, the psoriasis was gone!

I couldn't believe it! Mary couldn't believe it either, but she was certainly happy for me. It had taken me over ten years and about $750,000 to lick this thing . . . but I had finally won!

CHAPTER THREE

R⟨

YOUR JOURNEY

Chapter Three is where this becomes your journey. From this point forward, it's about your finding answers that will improve your health and prevent future sickness. Imagine having a practical diet that enables you to reset your system and to get rid of the foods that are causing inflammation. Talk about a breakthrough!

Don Colbert, MD

ANTI-INFLAMMATION LIVING

BY REMOVING THE TWO FOODS that were inflammatory for me, gluten and peppers, my body was able to heal.

I had my life back! It was a tremendous feeling, to know that I was free of the orange, asphalt-smelling coal tar that barely addressed my symptoms, but did absolutely nothing to address the root cause of my psoriasis.

Hope was birthed deep within me. It welled up, permeating my heart and mind with the belief that specific sicknesses could be addressed at the root level. And if it couldn't be cured, it usually could be controlled. I had to wonder what that would mean to me, to my patients, and to the world!

Sure, my world had changed. My new reality prohibited me from eating gluten and peppers. Could I live with these new parameters? Absolutely! I was alive once again.

Interestingly, after six months of no gluten or peppers, I tried a few bites of different peppers. No problem. A few days later, I tried a bit more. No side effects at all. I continue to eat peppers, but I learned to rotate them every few days. (Rotation is vital for those who reintroduce foods that were once inflammatory.) I don't eat peppers at every meal and I don't drink my salsa like I used to, but in moderation, peppers no longer bother me.

Not so with gluten. To this day, I have to avoid gluten. It brings the rash back. In the late 1990s, when I quit eating gluten, there were no restaurants that I knew of that were gluten free. I avoided breads, croutons, cookies, crackers, etc., but discovered that most sauces, salad dressings, and gravies still contained gluten. After unexpectedly breaking out many more times, I learned the hard way that many foods I thought were gluten free really were not. I have to follow my gluten-free diet very carefully, but I do not have celiac disease. Those who have celiac disease can actually die if they continue to eat gluten. (See "Appendix G: Gluten Is Everywhere" at the back of the book.)

HOW THIS AFFECTS US ALL

Looking back, my search for an answer to my psoriasis took me down some paths that were not that helpful, while other paths were extremely beneficial. Through it all, I can say that at least I was falling forward.

Then one day I hit my head against the foundation stone of food. It was both the answer and the problem, all at the same time.

I learned from firsthand experience—and have since then proven thousands of times with patients from around the world— that the root of most common diseases is due to inflammation from the foods we eat.

What did it mean to me? It meant healing when I applied this truth to my life.

What does it mean to you? It could be the difference between life and death, health and constant sickness, freedom and captivity.

The fact that food sensitivity causes inflammation is a reality that usually and eventually affects most of us. I knew diet was the factor that changed things for me. Still, the challenge I struggled with was that we medical doctors are taught to treat symptoms with medicines.

Suppose someone goes into a doctor's office with these symptoms:

- Abdominal bloating
- Headaches
- Cough
- Runny nose
- Feeling under the weather
- Stomachache
- Loose stools
- Hives

No doubt, the doctor will whip out his or her prescription pad and prescribe a medicine to address the symptoms. Interestingly, this is the exact list (from the Australian NSW Food Authority) of the most common symptoms of food intolerance.

In its simplest form, *food intolerance* is where our bodies usually lack a certain enzyme to digest a food. Being "lactose intolerant" is one such intolerance that people talk about all the time, and that means the body lacks the enzyme lactase to properly digest cow's milk. Almond milk, coconut milk, and rice milk are good substitutes.

Some say that a *food sensitivity* is a milder version of *food intolerance* and that a food "doesn't agree" with your gastrointestinal (GI) tract. This may be the case at the superficial level, but foods that cause inflammation are usually doing a lot more damage than we realize. With food sensitivities the inflammation doesn't usually flare up until hours or days later.

A *food allergy*, on the other hand, is where the body reacts strongly and usually immediately to a food, giving someone swollen lips, swollen tongue, hives, eczema, or even anaphylaxis. Inhalers, epinephrine, antihistamines, and steroids are usually needed to reverse the allergic reaction at this point. An allergic reaction to peanuts is a common food allergy. An increasingly common allergy is found in people who have celiac disease (allergic to gluten).

Much more could be said or explained about food allergies and food intolerances, but our focus here is food sensitivity. Why? Because I believe it is causing far more long-term health problems than food allergies and food intolerances combined.

Inflammation is the result of food sensitivities, and inflammation is at the root of almost every chronic disease.

> ## FACTOID
>
> According to US Centers for Disease Control, 90 percent of food allergies are associated with these eight food types:
>
> - Cow's milk
> - Hen's eggs
> - Peanuts
> - Soy foods
> - Wheat
> - Fish
> - Crustacean shellfish (shrimp, lobster, crab)
> - Tree nuts (almonds, cashews, walnuts, pecans, etc.)

INFLAMMATION IS CALLING

Inflammation has a very loud voice, and it is warning us to take action. We have been trained—both doctors and patients—to turn off the alarm, to treat symptoms and not the real problems.

That doesn't make the problem go away.

As you may know, there are two types of inflammation. The first is the "good" one. It is acute inflammation, such as you get with a sore throat, a splinter, or a sprained ankle. Your body is inflaming that specific place in your body to deal with your problem. The key factor is that it is on a short-term basis; white blood cells, antibodies, and other inflammatory mediators are sent to the area to fight the sickness (i.e., inflamed tonsils) or wall off the infection (i.e., splinter).

The "bad" type of inflammation is chronic inflammation and it is long-term, unrelenting, and invariably leads to disease. Let's say you have inflammation of the arteries and are not aware of it and/or do nothing to stop it. Consider this: Approximately 90 percent of all cardiovascular diseases are caused by inflammation!

Any food sensitivity is an inflammatory reaction, and when you continually eat foods that you are sensitive to, that eventually causes symptoms associated with inflammation and may eventually lead to disease. Ignoring the results is not going to bring health. It's doing the exact opposite. Consider:

- Chronic inflammation of the joints causes arthritis, and 90 percent of arthritis patients have osteoarthritis (chronic inflammation in the knees, back, neck, or fingers).
- Inflammation of the brain is associated with dementia, Alzheimer's disease, autism, schizophrenia and bipolar disorder.
- Inflammation in the arteries causes most cardiovascular diseases.
- Inflammation in the muscles causes fibromyalgia.
- Inflammation in the skin causes eczema and psoriasis.

My psoriasis, for example, was never going to go away on its own. As long as I kept eating the two key foods (gluten and peppers) that I was sensitive to—which then directly caused inflammation in my GI tract—which then caused inflammation in my skin—nothing was going to change.

> ### WISE BEVERAGE CHOICES
>
> - Water with lemon or lime (may add stevia)
> - Sparkling water
> - Tea (with stevia)
> - Coffee (with stevia) and coconut or almond milk

My inflammation was yelling at me, yet it took over ten years to answer that call. Thankfully, our bodies are made in such a way that they can heal quite rapidly once we have removed the "thorn" that is causing the inflammation.

Whatever your health-related "thorn" is, I would bet that inflammation is a part of it. And in all reality, if you ignore the voice of inflammation, will the ailment go away?

It probably won't. Plain and simple.

Can you live with your ailment? Yes, probably, but why settle for just surviving when you can thrive?

OTHER PIECES TO THE PUZZLE

I have come to see that when dealing with sickness caused by inflammation, there are often other factors that may play a part. With me, the trauma of my heatstroke and the heartbreak of my lawsuit were two such factors.

It would be very hard to prove that these factors caused the inflammation (usually it's the food that causes the inflammation), but these factors are connected in a very real way to the sickness itself. Here is what I've found:

With most diseases, there is usually an emotional trauma somewhere in the patient's past.

Admittedly, the world is full of sick and wounded people. We are all accustomed to seeing the sicknesses people carry on the outside, yet our emotions play such an important part in our sickness and subsequent health.

Because there are other pieces to the puzzle, I run more tests on my patients than most doctors. I first examine them conventionally, then I do numerous other lab and nutritional tests. I also do a comprehensive history and ask pages and pages of questions so that I have a very accurate picture of their dietary and lifestyle habits so we can tell why their health is what it is.

Connected to these other factors (i.e., my issue with the frivolous lawsuit) are related therapies that play a part in my patients' success. If there is pain, then it certainly needs to be dealt with. But unless these pains are dealt with properly, they will play a constant negative role in the lives of my patients.

Several years ago, I met with a pastor who was suffering from very high blood pressure. He was taking three different medications in an effort to try to control his out-of-control blood pressure. What surprised me was how he looked on the outside. He was soft spoken, not overweight at all,

UNWISE BEVERAGE CHOICES

- Soda (average 12-oz. soda has 10 tsp. of sugar)
- Lattes
- Sweet tea
- Alcohol
- Red Bull, Monster, and other energy drinks
- Large glasses of fruit juice (limit to 2 oz.)

he rode a Harley, was in his mid-50s, and was a very cool guy. He certainly didn't look the part.

As we worked through more of our preliminary questions (he was a new patient), I asked him, "How long have you had high blood pressure?"

"About five to six years," he replied.

I followed up, "Can you tell me about it?"

Immediately his ears turned red. Whatever he was about to say, I knew he was a hot reactor. Red ears are a signs of that. His blood pressure started going up.

He began to tell me his story. It involved betrayal (someone came in and took half of his congregation away) and loss (he eventually lost the church building itself). The more he talked, the redder he became. I checked his blood pressure and it was extremely high in spite of being on medication. He went from angry to hostile and the hostility was skyrocketing his blood pressure. Talk about pent-up emotions!

I took him through our trauma resolution therapy and forgiveness therapy, and during it he screamed one of the most blood-curdling screams I've ever heard. We prayed and he released it to the Lord. When he finished praying, he slumped over. I checked his blood pressure; it was totally normal. In the months that followed, we were able to wean him off two of his blood pressure medications. He was seething with anger and hostility, which was a perfect setup for a heart attack. Our forgiveness therapy and trauma resolution therapy were two pieces to his puzzle, a very important part, for he was hurting from a pain that no medication could touch.

In case you are wondering, I had to practice my own medicine and work through the process of forgiveness toward the woman who sued me, her attorney, and the news reporter. I had to deal with the trauma so that every time the mail came, my heart didn't leap out of my chest at the possibility of receiving another lawsuit. I'm over it now. I can talk about it. It's part of my own story.

Does time heal all wounds? No, contrary to what people might wish, time does *not* heal. Most people, this very instant, are carrying trauma around with them from events that occurred decades ago. I've seen patients who are so full of red-hot anger and resentment, pain and rage, you would think they had been hurt that very morning . . . only to find out it happened fifty years ago!

How can *that* be good for your body?

A person with heart disease feels they are one step from death. Fear, anger, and hostility can trigger heart attacks. On a practical level, they need to not sweat the small stuff. Practice forgiveness and let it go. Bitterness is not worth dying for!

If you are spending ten dollars' worth of energy for a two-cent problem, you are usually stressing your arteries. Instead of exploding or imploding, let it go. Emotions like hostility, frustration, and irritability are all connected with anger in some way, and that usually leads to heart disease. Just let it go!

Keep resentment under the radar and you see OCD (obsessive-compulsive disorder), PTSD (post-traumatic stress disorder), depression, high blood pressure, decreased immune function, heart disease, cancer, and autoimmune disease increase among the population . . . exactly what we see today!

Massive trauma, whether it is physical (like my heatstroke) or related (such as the tragic death of a loved one) can also cause a lot of internal pain and eventual disease. Part of what I do, in addition to forgiveness therapy, is to help remove the traumas that are plaguing my patients. This trauma resolution therapy can play a big part in setting the stage for eventual physical health.

We can even break the cravings for certain foods. When we are done, they are usually disgusted with the very foods that they craved just minutes before.

But the focus of this book is diet and health. My advice is to deal with your past. Resolve the trauma. Forgive. Move forward. No, it's not instant. It will take time, but it is worth it!

I don't know what happened to the woman who sued me, but that really doesn't matter. I am free of the anger and resentment. My point is, let those who have hurt you reap the rewards of their own life choices. You must choose to be free, for in that choice there is life, restoration, and health!

Back to the subject of inflammation . . . If you are wondering if you are suffering from inflammation from the foods you eat, I would say the answer is usually a resounding "Yes!"

That does not mean that you can see it or even feel it. Remember, the ultimate goal is both health *and* prevention. That is the journey we are all on.

IN SEARCH OF AN ANTI-INFLAMMATORY DIET

When I was in residency, I worked at weight loss centers on the weekends. I would help people lose weight, but usually they gained it right back. So many diets and fads came and went.

It was during that time that I first met Dr. Atkins (of the Atkins Diet). He was a diet "guru" back then, but sadly he died in 2003 from a fall on an icy New York City sidewalk. Debate rages to this day as to whether his history of heart attack, congestive heart failure, and hypertension were related to his diet or not. I had to wonder if those excessive animal proteins and fats were largely responsible for his heart disease.

I didn't know it at the time, but what I needed when I had full-blown, unchecked psoriasis was an anti-inflammatory diet. That makes good sense now, but it took years for the realization to sink in. And if an anti-inflammatory diet would have helped me, it would also be of tremendous benefit to my patients.

Over time, from studies, testing, trial and error, experience, and tracking my own patients, I learned that a person following an anti-inflammatory diet must:

- Eliminate sugars and sweets, or include very little
- Only eat small amounts of meat: 3–6 oz. once/twice a day (3–4 oz. for women, 3–6 oz. for men)
- Limit red meat to 3–6 oz. once/twice a week, or eliminate completely
- Follow a mostly plant-based diet
- Eliminate processed meats (hot dogs, salami, pepperoni, bacon, sausage, etc.)
- Include healthy starches with a low glycemic value, such as steel-cut oats, quinoa, beans, peas, lentils, sweet potatoes, etc.
- Avoid fried food
- Limit, avoid, or rotate every four days: pork, lamb, and shrimp, crab, lobster, or other shellfish
- Include healthy fats from macadamia nuts, cashews, walnuts, almonds, extra-virgin olive oil, and avocados
- Minimize intake of omega-6 fats (corn oil, safflower oil, sunflower oil, cotton seed oil, soybean oil)

- Include wild salmon (probably the highest anti-inflammatory food on the planet) and other wild, low-mercury fish
- Eliminate trans fats or hydrogenated fats
- Include extra-virgin olive oil
- Eliminate, limit, or rotate every four days grains (use legumes: beans, peas, lentils)
- Reach a healthy body weight because obesity is connected to most diseases today
- Minimize night shades (peppers, tomatoes, potatoes, paprika, eggplant) or rotate every four days
- Be able to improve, or control, type 2 diabetes
- Include exercise five days a week and balance your hormones
- Cope with stress
- Include more sleep
- Eliminate or limit GMO foods (most soy, corn, canola oil, and cottonseed oil)

I realized that the more I studied, tweaked, and revised this anti-inflammatory list, the more I was looking at the beginning of a healthy lifestyle that both treats and prevents most diseases.

That is something I could get excited about, something that would set a lot of people free. Imagine how entire families, populations, states, and even countries could be impacted. When a single chronic disease is said to have the potential to bankrupt the US Medicare system in the coming years, the financial benefits of being able to just control that one disease, let alone cure it, would be off the charts.

But it will require us to change.

I went to a seminar years ago with Mary at a massive hotel. At the event, there was a huge buffet section of fruits, salmon, grapes, vegetables, melons, whole grains, oatmeal, etc. On the other side of the room, there were mountains of bacon, sausage, gravy, waffles, donuts, pastries, etc. We watched as people lined up to eat. The alert, active, energetic, healthy people were in line for living foods, while the people who looked tired, bent over, sour in appearance, and with no spring in their step were lined up for the dead food. It was amazing to watch.

> ## FACTOID
>
> Inflammation is the root cause of most chronic diseases.

Sadly, most dead foods are highly inflammatory. And that makes it all about the choices we make. Without question, we need to be pursuing that which brings us health and helps us avoid disease. Health is the ideal long-term goal.

What I needed was an anti-inflammatory diet that would break the cycle. It had to be a diet that most patients could use as a foundational starting point for better health. It would need to be both informative as well as practical.

Based on what I have found, after decades of medical practice, research, study, and serving thousands of patients, these are the key components of the anti-inflammatory diet.

THE ANTI-INFLAMMATORY DIET

1. All vegetables three servings a day and more if able
   a. Steam, stir-fry, cook under low heat, or eat raw
   b. Vegetable soups, non-cream based. Homemade is best and you may add some organic meat
2. Meats: 3–4 oz. once/twice a day for women, 3–6 oz. once/twice a day for men

   a. Turkey (skinless), free-range chicken (skinless, white meat), or eggs (organic or free-range omega-3 eggs as well)

   b. When grilling, slice meat thin, marinate in red wine, pomegranate juice, cherry juice, or curry sauce, and remove all char from meat

   c. Eggs once/twice a week, only 1 yolk and 2–3 whites

   d. Avoid red meat or minimize to 3–6 oz. once or twice a week

3. Low mercury fish (see Appendix C for mercury levels of fish)
4. Fruits: at least two servings a day

   a. Berries, Granny Smith apples, lemon, and lime are low glycemic

   b. May eat all fruit but avoid fruit syrup and minimize dried fruit and fruit juice

5. Beans, peas, lentils (and other legumes), hummus: ½–2 cups daily, preferably before meals

   a. Bean soup, black bean, lentil, etc., prior to lunch and dinner

6. Raw nuts and seeds: almonds, hazelnuts, pecans, cashews, walnuts, macadamia nuts (at least one handful a day)
7. Salads with extra-virgin olive oil and vinegar (may use less olive oil and more vinegar if trying to lose weight); start with large salad with lunch and dinner (without croutons)
8. Dairy: low-fat dairy without sugar, such as Greek yogurt, low-fat cottage cheese
9. Starches: sweet potatoes, new potatoes, brown/wild rice, millet bread, brown rice pasta (use in moderation when choosing starches and at most only one serving per meal and limit to size of a tennis ball for women and 1–2 tennis balls for

men), and minimize or avoid corn unless it is non-GMO and not processed. Minimize or avoid gluten, but may use sprouted bread (Ezekiel 4:9 bread) in moderation, if you are not obese or suffering from any disease.

10. Oils: 2–4 tablespoons of extra-virgin olive oil daily (can be put on salads) and can use more if not overweight or obese

11. Vinegar (any type): 2–4 tablespoons or more daily or as desired

12. Drinks:
    a. Alkaline water or sparking water (may add lemon or lime)
    b. Green, black, white tea (may add lemon or lime) with stevia
    c. Coffee with coconut milk and stevia (if desired)
    d. Low-fat coconut milk or almond milk in place of regular milk
    e. Pomegranate juice: 2 oz. daily
    f. No sugar [use stevia or lohan (monk fruit) guo or erythritol to sweeten]
    g. No cream (use low-fat coconut milk)

13. Avoid:
    a. All gluten (wheat, barley, rye, spelt, pasta, crackers, bagels, pretzels, most cereal, etc.; see Appendix F: Gluten Is Everywhere)
    b. Organ meats if obese or suffering from chronic diseases
    c. Sugar
    d. All fried foods
    e. All processed foods
    f. High-glycemic foods: white rice, instant potatoes, etc.
    g. GMO foods, such as most corn, soy, canola oil, and cottonseed oil.
    h. Inflammatory meats such as shellfish, pork, lamb, veal,

and red meats (avoid completely or rotate every 4 days or longer, and limit amount to 3–6 oz.)

14. Rotate vegetables and meats every four days (do not eat the same foods every day); for example, on day 1 eat chicken; day 2, turkey; day 3, salmon; and so on

15. Organic: Choose organic as much as possible, but it's still a healthy diet even if you can't do organic. With a healthy body, eating non-organic is fine. (See Appendix B for Clean Fifteen [produce with minimal pesticides] and Dirty Dozen [produce with highest pesticide residues].)

I have had hundreds of patients over the years go on this anti-inflammatory diet, and the results have been astounding. But it is really nothing more than removing the food sources of inflammation and then letting the body reboot, similar to rebooting a computer.

Not long ago, a mother called and made an appointment for me to see her six-year-old autistic daughter. The nearest appointment was set for two months out, and before we concluded the call, the mother asked me, "Is there anything I can do to prepare for the visit?"

FACTOID

Diseases are related to our diets. I have found it's always food-related.

Knowing I would introduce her to this anti-inflammatory diet, but only after doing all the usual screenings and testing I do, I told my nurse to tell the mother to begin by removing just two things from her daughter's diet: wheat and dairy.

When I finally saw them at their scheduled appointment, the patient's mother was ecstatic. When she calmed down, she explained, "My daughter is already at least 50 percent better!"

Her daughter was already experiencing at least a 50 percent improvement, and they had technically not even started the anti-inflammatory diet yet.

Not bad . . . not bad at all!

CHAPTER FOUR

R

YOUR JOURNEY

Chapter Four outlines the super-healthy Mediterranean Diet. You will discover several raw ingredients that may have negatively been affecting your health, and why. From there it builds into what I believe is the world's best anti-inflammatory diet. This is the future—your future!—we are talking about. This is exciting!

Don Colbert, MD

THE BEST DIET FOR HEALTH AND PREVENTION OF DISEASE

BACK IN THE EARLY 1990s when Bob came to me, he was only forty-five years old, but he already had a history of hypertension, high triglycerides, high cholesterol, type 2 diabetes, and obesity. He stood 5'8" tall and weighed 275 pounds. He was taking medications for each of his health problems.

He loved his donuts and coffee for breakfast, a burger and fries with a soda for lunch, and a large pizza or burrito for dinner, with a big bowl of ice cream at bedtime.

One day, I received a call from the emergency room at a local hospital. Bob had just survived a massive heart attack.

After he was released, we talked further and he decided that no food was worth dying for. He had two teenage sons and a young daughter and he wanted to be around when they grew up, graduated from high school and college, and got married.

I worked with him on his diet, part of which included getting off sugar, burgers, pizza, ice cream, and all fast food. He also started exercising. All told, he lost one hundred pounds that year! By the time he reached 175 pounds, he was off all of his medications.

Bob was a great example of what every patient needs: a

long-term, healthy lifestyle diet. The yo-yo effect of trying a diet, losing and regaining the weight, then trying another diet, is rarely effective long term, not to mention the fact that the diet itself may not be healthy. A diet high in meat proteins or dairy or wheat or even vegetables (if you are sensitive to them) is not necessarily going to be good for your body. It goes back to the inflammation that we all need to avoid or minimize.

What we need is a lifestyle of eating that is anti-inflammatory and good for your long-term health and prevention of disease. That would be a diet worth sticking to.

Like you, I see diets come and go. Some of them are strange, others are unhealthy, and some are downright dangerous. Many, however, are a good step in the right direction.

But still, I needed a healthy diet that would truly bring health to my patients and that they could follow long-term for the rest of their lives. Treating and re-treating their symptoms could never be the answer. Anti-inflammatory food was—and is—the foundation of their healing.

The best diet I found (in the 1990s and early 2000) was the Mediterranean Diet. I've studied all the diets, but even the Mediterranean Diet is not entirely anti-inflammatory. I'll explain that later, but first, we need to understand just what makes the Mediterranean Diet so effective.

THE MEDITERRANEAN DIET

The Mediterranean Diet, like the typical "health" pyramid the USDA produces, is built on levels or layers, where you eat the most of the food items at the bottom of the pyramid and the least of the food items at the top. With that in mind, here is how the Mediterranean Diet looks, from the bottom up:

Level One: complex carbohydrates in the form of brown rice, whole-grain rice, whole-grain pasta, and whole-grain bread (the fresher the better). Other possible options include cracked whole wheat (bulgur wheat), couscous, course cornmeal (polenta), and potatoes.

Level Two: fruits, vegetables, nuts, beans, and other legumes. Salads are made of dark green leafy lettuce, fresh vine-ripened tomatoes, broccoli, spinach, peppers, onions, and cucumbers. The vegetables are often mixed with pasta or rice, used in salads, served as appetizers, or offered as a main or side dish. Fruits are at this level, but are usually a dessert or snack. Nuts are toppings to add flavor and texture. The beans and legumes are usually in soups, added to salads, used as dips (i.e., hummus), or as a main dish.

Level Three: olive oil, used instead of other oils, butter, margarine, etc. Not only for cooking, it is commonly mixed with balsamic vinegar as a salad dressing.

Level Four: cheese and yogurt, in small amounts. Freshly grated Parmesan on pasta or a little feta cheese on a salad is common. Yogurt (about a cup a day) is how milk is usually eaten, and it is low fat or nonfat, usually served with fresh fruit added. Yogurt is also a salad dressing (i.e., mixed with dill, garlic, onion, and cucumbers).

> ### REVELATION
> Eating quickly means your brain registers full . . . but after you have already eaten too much.

Level Five: fish, eaten more than other meats, in about 4-ounce portions several times a week.

Level Six: chicken, turkey, and eggs. Chicken in 3- to 6-ounce portions a few times a week is common. The meat is usually skinless and added to soups, stews, and other dishes loaded with vegetables. Only 1 to 4 eggs per week.

Level Seven: red meat, in the form of beef, veal, pork, sheep, lamb, and goats, is eaten only a few times a month. It is then often served as a topping to a vegetable, pasta, or rice dish.

The Mediterranean Diet is of course supposed to mirror what those in the Mediterranean actually eat. Most meals are served with a glass of red wine or bottled water.

What you have just read is more than just a diet. It is a way of life or a lifestyle. And if you were to investigate, you would find that these people in the Mediterranean countries do not usually have a membership to a local gym. They usually walk everywhere, including to work. As for eating, it's a big affair, with conversation and laughter, and they take their time. We in America scarf down our food, typically in less than ten minutes and often while driving or while watching TV.

Maybe you had a grandmother who said, "Slow down and chew your food!" Those were not just wasted words. It is very good advice, and it is something that naturally happens when you enjoy a dinner with others. Chewing your food thirty times is the best for digestion and food absorption. Try it the next time you are eating. If you are chowing down, slow down and you will probably feel better and have significantly less indigestion and heartburn.

> **FACTOID**
>
> stevia is a natural substitute for sugar, and it has no harmful side effects.

Eating at a slower pace, with friends and family, not only helps you control your appetite, but it also helps reduce your stress. Nothing wrong with that!

IMPLEMENTING THE MEDITERRANEAN DIET

If you want to shift over to the Mediterranean Diet, then there are thirteen important steps to take. Some steps and decisions will be easier than others, but every single step is a good one, except with certain grains. Here is what it usually takes:

1. Eliminate processed foods, which include chips, snacks made with hydrogenated fat, cakes, candies, cookies, crackers, high sugar cereals, white bread, high-processed foods, and high sugar foods.
2. Substitute olive oil for butter, margarine, salad dressings, and other oils. Get rid of other oils, salad dressings, lard, Crisco, and other products with hydrogenated fat.
3. Buy only whole grain items, fresh fruits, fresh vegetables, nuts, and seeds.
4. Cook and bake with whole grain products.
5. Avoid fried or deep-fried foods.
6. Choose low-fat, plain yogurt, and sweeten with stevia or fresh fruit.
7. Limit cheese to small amounts of Parmesan or feta mixed with salads or main dishes.
8. Buy fish and poultry more than red meat.
9. Eat red meat very sparingly.
10. Cut out sugary sweets.
11. Enjoy a glass of red wine (caution: may lead to dependence or alcoholism) or sparkling water with lunch or dinner.

12. Walk, bike, and run as much as you can.

13. Slow down and enjoy your dining experience.

TAKING THINGS TO THE NEXT LEVEL

A few years ago, a rigorous study (conducted by Dr. Ramon Estruch, a professor of medicine at the University of Barcelona, and his colleagues[2]) spanning several years found that the Mediterranean Diet reduced the chances of strokes, heart attacks, and deaths due to heart disease by an astounding 30 percent! They actually stopped the study early because those who were not on the Mediterranean Diet were found to be at such a high risk that they felt it was unethical to keep them from the diet.

That alone is a good enough reason to be on the diet. For many years, I have plugged my patients in to this diet, with similar great results. It's very gratifying to be able, as a doctor, to give patients a practical and effective way to treat many of their ailments long-term. Prescribing a medication that only treats the symptoms is so superficial.

> ### HEALTH
>
> Dr. William Davis notes, "So this is your brain on wheat: Digestion yields morphine-like compounds that bind to the brain's opiate receptors. It induces a form of reward."[3] It sounds like we may very well be addicted to our gluten!

But is there more? Am I missing something? Can I do better? I always wonder that, and I should as a medical doctor.

The more patients I treated, especially those from the United States, the more I realized that something was wrong with their diet. Actually, it was not the diet at all . . . it was the food itself.

Inflammation was still getting through to my patients. I knew what it was, but it took years to confirm my findings. Other doctors have also come forward with their findings, and it confirmed my hunch.

The Mediterranean Diet is still an incredibly healthy diet, but I've found the need to modify it. Why? Because the raw ingredients of today are not what they used to be. That may sound a little odd, but in its simplest form:

Most grains and corns have been crossbred, hybridized, or genetically modified.

Dr. William Davis, in his best-selling book, *Wheat Belly*, does an incredible job explaining the changes to wheat and how that affects us today. He says:

Wheat naturally evolved to only a modest degree over the centuries, but it has changed dramatically in the past fifty years under the influence of agricultural scientists. Wheat strains have been hybridized, crossbred, and introgressed to make the wheat plant resistant to environmental conditions, such as drought, or pathogens, such as fungi. But most of all, genetic changes have been induced to increase yield per acre. The average yield on a modern North American farm is more than tenfold greater than farms of a century ago.[4]

And what does it matter? In the health and medical world, it matters for one huge reason: *inflammation*.

What was created to feed the poor and grow faster and need less irrigation and be hearty is no doubt an engineering marvel! But it is this genetic recoding of the wheat that brings about the effects I see in the doctor's office.

In addition to the revised gluten creating inflammation, there are other side effects. Davis also explained how other studies with gluten have found that it can be addictive and many people have withdrawal symptoms when they go without wheat. It also increases your appetite. Not good at all, and I see that all the time coming through my office doors in many shapes and sizes.

And when you talk about diabetes, consider the fact that nutritionists more than thirty years ago found that wheat increases blood sugar more than table sugar! You can see why even the whole wheat bread of the Mediterranean Diet, though it is better than white bread, is still creating havoc among patients who are fighting obesity, diabetes, hypertension, high cholesterol, and a host of other ailments.

> ## TRENDING
>
> The most commonly eaten foods in America are white bread, coffee, and hot dogs.

The effect of the daily recommended amount of whole grains on my diabetic patients was a good enough reason for me to deviate away from the industry standard. I have had patients check their blood sugars before eating grains, even corn, and then an hour later see their sugar levels spike 70–120 mg/dl (milligrams per decileter) higher than their starting levels. That causes a dramatic release of insulin, similar to that of eating sugar. (If you are wondering, non-diabetic sugar levels would usually go up only about 20 to 40 points in comparison.)

Staying on the "eat 6–10 servings a day of bread, cereal, pasta, rice" as the government recommends was not an option anyway. I started modifying the diets of my diabetic patients years ago for this very reason.

The gluten craze is not really for the very small percentage of people who are truly allergic to gluten. I find it very interesting that "as many as 40 percent of us can't properly process gluten," says Dr. David Perlmutter in his best-selling book, *Grain Brain.*

The altered (crossbred, hybridized) gluten is wreaking havoc on our health. It really is. And it is exactly that inflammation that causes so much trouble. Why? Because every single degenerative disease has inflammation as the foundation. *Every single one of them!*

When I work with ADHD, ADD, autistic, bipolar, and schizophrenic patients, inflammation also comes directly into play. Dr. Perlmutter points out that "gluten, and a high-carbohydrate diet for that matter, are among the most prominent stimulators of inflammatory pathways that reach the brain."

> ### HEALTH
>
> Dr. Perlmutter asks, "What if we're all sensitive to gluten from the perspective of the brain?"[5] That is a very good question!

Wow!

Interestingly, back in 1994, the American Diabetes Association stated that Americans should get 60–70 percent of their calories from carbohydrates. Guess what happened to the number of patients with diabetes? Yes, it went through the roof! But here is where that stat really takes things to the next level: as Dr. Perlmutter notes, "Becoming a diabetic doubles your risk of Alzheimer's disease."

As for corn, the number one crop in the United States, 88 percent of it is GMO (genetically modified organism). These plants have had their DNA altered in a laboratory by genes from other plants, even animals, viruses, or bacteria.

It isn't just corn that is genetically modified. Cottonseed oil (94 percent of what we grow is GMO), soy (93 percent), canola oil (90 percent), papaya (75 percent of Hawaiian papaya), and sugar beets (90 percent, and more than half of sugar sold in the United States comes from sugar beets) are just a few of our staples that are not what they used to be.

It is estimated that between 70 and 85 percent of processed foods that we find in our local grocery stores contain GMO ingredients. The FDA does not require labels to inform you of GMOs in your food, so technically there is no way to be sure of the exact percentage that we consume. Other GMO foods include tomatoes, potatoes, squash, golden rice, animal feed, and even farm-raised salmon.

As you can see, grains and corn, among other raw ingredients, are not even close to what they used to be! One chief side effect of these alterations is the inflammation they cause in our bodies, and I see that on a daily basis.

The best way to avoid GMO foods is to avoid processed foods and/or choose organic foods. Organic foods are not genetically modified.

Coming back to the Mediterranean Diet, I couldn't believe what Dr. Perlmutter wrote. He makes it plain when he states:

If you modify the traditional Mediterranean Diet by removing all gluten-containing foods and limiting sugary fruits and non-gluten carbs, you have yourself the perfect grain-brain-free diet.

Exactly! That is what I have been saying for years and that is the most exciting part of this book. You will soon see in the following chapters how the modified Mediterranean Diet can usually and effectively treat (cure, control, or manage) every major disease.

WHAT DO YOU CRAVE?

The deeper I dug into health and nutrition—trying to treat the cause of a sickness rather than treat just the symptoms—I began to come across similarities that seemed to be repetitive. (Naturally, if it helps my patients, I'll keep track of it.)

Interestingly, when it comes to food, our bodies often crave the very food that we love . . . but should hate. Our bodies want the very foods that are making us sick.

> **HEALTH**
>
> Choose organic to avoid GMOs, especially with corn and soy.

Maybe it's our minds playing tricks on us, but whatever the case . . . if you are craving something, take a second look at it; you may want to find out why.

Consider the following cravings that I have noticed and tracked for years with my patients:

- *Sugar*: Usually craved by those with diabetes, cancer, ADHD, Alzheimer's, obesity

- *Dairy*: Usually craved by those with ear/sinus troubles, autism, osteoarthritis, IBS (irritable bowel syndrome), Crohn's disease
- *Refined grains*: Usually craved by those with obesity, diabetes, dementia, ADD, ADHD, autism, hypertension, high cholesterol
- *Corn and wheat*: Usually craved by those with dementia, autism, ADHD, IBS (irritable bowel syndrome), diabetes, obesity, autoimmune disease
- *MSG/artificial sweeteners*: Usually craved by those with migraines, seizures, memory loss, bipolar disorder, ADHD, ADD, obesity
- *Deep fried foods*: Usually craved by those with heart disease, vascular disease, obesity, arthritis, hypertension, high cholesterol
- *Trans fats/hydrogenated oils* (cake icing, most commercial peanut butter): Usually craved by those with dementia, Alzheimer's, heart disease, cancer, hypertension, high cholesterol
- *Red meat/pork*: Usually craved by those with osteoarthritis, breast cancer, prostate cancer, cardiovascular disease, hypertension, high cholesterol
- *Milk shakes, pizza, hot dogs*: Usually craved by those with ADHD, ADD, autism, arthritis, obesity, diabetes, hypertension, high cholesterol

I'm not saying if you crave a hamburger that you have or will have breast cancer or if you crave a pizza that you have or will have ADD. What I am saying is that a lot of my patients with certain diseases had these similar food cravings. It's something to think about.

If your health would improve by letting go of what you crave, would it be worth it? I have had many patients who suffered from migraines get off MSG (monosodium glutamate) and artificial sweeteners and in a matter of weeks their headaches were gone. For them, the craving for food with MSG (i.e., usually found in Korean, Japanese, and Chinese food) is simply something they should resist.

Definitely food for thought!

THE *MODIFIED* MEDITERRANEAN DIET

How exactly did we modify the already great Mediterranean Diet to turn it into the best anti-inflammatory diet in the world? In a nutshell, avoid, minimize, or rotate every four days the wheat, and corn.

That may seem like a minor alteration, but it's actually a huge shift, one that is bringing healing to thousands of people!

Without further ado, here is the modified Mediterranean Diet:

Level #1: fruits, vegetables, nuts, beans, and other legumes. Salads consist of dark green leafy lettuce, fresh vine-ripened tomatoes, broc-

> ### HEALTH RISKS POSED BY GENETIC ENGINEERING[7]
> 1. Toxicity
> 2. Allergic reactions
> 3. Antibiotic resistance
> 4. Immuno-suppression
> 5. Cancer
> 6. Loss of Nutrition

coli, spinach, peppers, onions, and cucumbers. Serve vegetables in salads, as appetizers, or as a main or side dish. Fruits are usually a dessert or snack. Use nuts as toppings to add flavor and texture. The beans and legumes are usually in soups, added to salads, used as dips (i.e., hummus), or as a main dish.

Level #2: steel-cut oats and quinoa, millet or millet bread, brown rice, and sweet potatoes. If you are not gluten sensitive, trying to lose weight, or suffering from high blood pressure, diabetes, high cholesterol, or another inflammatory disease, then potatoes, sprouted bread (i.e., Ezekiel 4:9 bread), or fermented bread (i.e., sourdough bread) are fine on occasion, rotated every four days, and with moderation (the size of a tennis ball for women and 1-2 tennis balls for men).

OPTIONS

Fermenting, sprouting, or soaking removes some of the inflammatory components of wheat. Thus, sprouted wheat bread, Ezekiel 4:9 bread, and sourdough bread are less inflammatory. Instead of eliminating wheat, if one is not obese or suffering from any disease, you may eat it every four days. Even non-GMO corn kernels or corn on the cob every four days with moderation is okay.

Level #3: olive oil, used instead of other oils, including butter, margarine, etc. Not only for cooking, it is commonly mixed with balsamic vinegar as a salad dressing.

Level #4: cheese and yogurt, in small amounts. Freshly grated Parmesan on pasta or a little feta cheese on a salad is common. Yogurt (about a cup) is how milk is usually eaten, and it is low fat or nonfat, served with fresh fruit added. Yogurt may also be used as a salad dressing (i.e., mixed with dill, garlic, onion, and cucumbers). Many of my patients are sensitive to dairy and thus may need to minimize, avoid, or rotate it every four days.

Level #5: fish, eaten more than other meats, in about 4- to 6-ounce portions several times a week. Choose low-mercury fish (see Appendix C).

Level #6: chicken, turkey, and eggs. Chicken in 3- to 6-ounce portions a few times a week is common. The meat is usually skinless and added to soups, stews, and other dishes loaded with vegetables. Only 2 to 6 eggs per week. I recommend 1 yolk/3 whites as egg ratio.

Level #7: red meat, in the form of beef, veal, pork, sheep, lamb, and goat, is eaten in 3- to 6-ounce portions once or twice a week or just a few times a month. It is then often served as a topping to a vegetable, pasta, or rice dish.

Visually, with the most and biggest at the bottom and the least and smallest at the top, it looks like this:

```
          #7
        #6#6
       #5#5#5
      #4#4#4#4
     #3#3#3#3#3
    #2#2#2#2#2#2
   #1#1#1#1#1#1#1
```

The modified Mediterranean Diet is the best anti-inflammatory diet in the world, but of course, if you are allergic or sensitive to a food (i.e., peanuts, dairy, or fish), then don't eat it. Your revised version has then become your own slightly modified Mediterranean Diet.

It is this very diet—with a few minor adjustments, like avoiding food cravings that lean toward a certain ailment—that is so effective in treating specific illnesses. Quite literally, this modified Mediterranean Diet can usually effectively cure, control, or manage every major disease.

That is a pretty bold statement, but as you will see in the coming chapters, it is also happening!

Not long ago a man from a Central American country contacted me. He was suffering from type 2 diabetes and severely high blood pressure. He was also obese. According to the customs, he ate corn at every meal, with lots of rice and meat. I told him right away, "Keep the beans, avocados, and lentils, but get rid of the rest."

Corn chips were out, but lentil chips or bean chips would work. Lettuce wraps, with chicken, onions, and avocados, were also a good option for him, as was hummus and olive oil with celery sticks, which is good to curb the hunger yet high in good fats, protein, and fiber while low in sugars.

Within months, both his blood sugar levels (he tested his HbA1C number every three months) and his high blood pressure

---

HEALTH

The average American gets 6.9 hours of sleep a night. Too little sleep increases the risk for heart disease, obesity, type 2 diabetes, dementia, accelerated aging, fatigue, depression, and a compromised immune system. We need seven to eight hours a night, consistently.

---

came down beautifully, and he lost a lot of weight. He emails us regularly, but he has successfully controlled his diabetes and his high blood pressure already.

Like I said, this is where things get really interesting!

CHAPTER FIVE

℞

YOUR JOURNEY

Chapter Five is amazing! It outlines the most practical and effective way to both lose weight and keep it off. Since so many diseases are directly related to obesity, getting this under your belt is an absolute must for your ongoing health and lifestyle. Over the years, I have had thousands of patients apply this, with amazing results!

Don Colbert, MD

LOSING WEIGHT FOR GOOD

WHEN SALLY WALKED THROUGH my office doors, I knew we were talking about more than weight loss . . . which is usually the case. Being overweight or obese multiplies your risks for thirty-five major diseases, including but not limited to:

- Type 2 diabetes
- Heart disease
- Stroke
- Arthritis
- Hypertension
- Acid reflux
- Sleep apnea
- Alzheimer's disease
- Infertility
- Erectile dysfunction
- Gallbladder disease
- Many different cancers
- . . . and much more!

I'll skip to the good part right away: she lost more than seventy pounds and has kept it off! She also completely took control over her other ailments.

She started with the modified Mediterranean Diet, then focused on the portion and timing of her meals—all in addition to more exercise and a positive mental attitude. She was the one who did all the work, and she deserves credit for her effort and choices.

The point is, she did what it took, and if you need to lose weight, so can you.

WHERE DID THIS WEIGHT COME FROM?

Is the extra weight biological? Sure, some of it might be our genes or our metabolism. It could even be the result of emotional eating, which is where people try to "deal with" a stress, crisis, anxiety, loneliness, or some other factor by eating food. This never works.

Most likely, however, part of our weight problem is due to lack of exercise. Our society as a whole, from children to adults, requires less and less physical exercise to get things done. The more technologically advanced we seem to get, the less physical we become, and that is evidenced by our expanding waistlines.

Sometimes it's our own family members who slow us down. When I ask my patients (75 percent are women) if they are willing to change their diets, many say "no" due to their kids or their husbands. The fact is, if family members won't help with the person's desire to change, it's going to be tough. I've tracked it. Sadly, 30–40 percent of the time, the spouse is sabotaging the patient's efforts to make better choices and get well! Every patient needs a support group, so if your family isn't there for you, find a local neighborhood support group, church support group, or online group.

Another common reason for weight gain is stress. Excessive stress messes with our cortisol levels (bringing on the toxic belly fat), our appetite hormones, and may trigger food addictions. Learn to chill out!

Another probability is the way we eat. We consume too much sweet, processed, fried, packaged, boxed, artificial food. In fact, it's downright scary. According to the USDA, the average American consumes anywhere between 150 to 170 pounds of refined sugars each year![8]

It could also be the result of the wheat and corn that we are eating, as you have already read in the previous chapter. Wheat, corn, and GMO foods can cause a host of health and hormonal issues, which promote weight gain.

One reason we struggle with weight is because food companies are so incredibly talented at making food so irresistible to the five senses that we may become addicted to it. They hire the brightest minds, including food chemists, psychologists, and marketers, to make their food so attractive that we can't eat just one!

CRAVINGS

The University of Illinois did a study that found Americans' favorite comfort foods are:

- Potato chips
- Ice cream
- Cookies
- Chocolate
- Pizza or pasta

The unwanted weight can also come with our culture and family upbringing. I was raised in Mississippi and my mom cooked traditional Southern food with biscuits and gravy or corn bread; almost everything was fried; and dessert went with every dinner, along with sweet tea. Many family members died of heart attacks, strokes, and other diseases associated with obesity. One uncle had both of his legs amputated at age sixty due to diabetes, but was obese for years before diabetes set in.

According to the CDC (Centers for Disease Control and Prevention), about 70 percent of adults are overweight and over 35 percent are obese. Those numbers are only increasing. From 1980 to 2000, obesity rates doubled among adults, doubled among children, and tripled among adolescents.

And as the national obesity rates increase, so do our national rates of thirty-five major diseases. I have been practicing medicine for over thirty years, have written many books on weight loss, and have treated thousands of patients for weight loss. To sum it up into one sentence, I would say this: *The main behaviors causing the obesity epidemic are preventable!*

What are those main behaviors that can be prevented? They are:

1. bad food choices
2. bad beverage choices
3. physical inactivity

We can, therefore, overcome obesity by doing the very opposite:

1. good food choices
2. good beverage choices
3. physical activity

Yes, it's pretty simple. And it will take work, effort, and commitment, but isn't your health worth it?

WHERE WEIGHT LOSS BEGINS

I start weight-loss patients with the healthy lifestyle diet of the modified Mediterranean Diet. It is not only the foundation to good health, but it is a lifestyle they can follow for years and years to come, which means their weight loss will be a permanent fixture rather than a passing fad. We begin here:

Level #1: fruits, vegetables, nuts, beans, and other legumes. Salads consist of dark green leafy lettuce, fresh vine-ripened tomatoes, broccoli, spinach, peppers, onions, and cucumbers. Serve vegetables in salads, as appetizers, or as a main or side dish. Fruits are usually a dessert or snack. Use nuts as toppings to add flavor and texture. The beans and legumes are usually in soups, added to salads, used as dips (i.e., hummus), or as a main dish.

Level #2: steel-cut oats and quinoa, millet or millet bread, brown rice, and sweet potatoes. If you are not gluten sensitive, trying to lose weight, or suffering from high blood pressure, diabetes, or high cholesterol, then potatoes, sprouted bread (i.e., Ezekiel 4:9 bread), or fermented bread (i.e., sourdough bread) are fine on occasion; rotate it every four days and with moderation.

Level #3: olive oil used instead of other vegetable oils, butter, margarine, etc. Not only for cooking, it is commonly mixed with balsamic vinegar as a salad dressing.

Level #4: cheese and yogurt, in small amounts. Freshly grated Parmesan on pasta or a little feta cheese on a salad is common. Yogurt (about a cup) is how milk is usually eaten, and it is low fat or nonfat, served with fresh fruit added. Yogurt can also be used in a salad dressing (i.e., mixed with dill, garlic, onion, and cucumbers). Dairy may need to be rotated every four days.

Level #5: fish, eaten more than other meats, in about 4- to 6-ounce portions several times a week.

Level #6: chicken, turkey, and eggs. Chicken in 3- to 6-ounce portions a few times a week is common. The meat is usually skinless and added to soups, stews, and other dishes loaded with vegetables. Only 2 to 6 eggs per week. I recommend 1 yolk/3 whites as an egg ratio.

Level #7: red meat, in the form of beef, veal, pork, sheep, lamb, and goat, is eaten in 3- to 6-ounce portions only one to two times a week, often served as a topping to a vegetable, pasta, or rice dish.

With that as the foundation, the three main behaviors of good food choices, good beverage choices, and physical activity don't look nearly so challenging, do they? Much more doable!

```
            PORTIONS

               #7
             #6#6
           #5#5#5
         #4#4#4#4
       #3#3#3#3#3
     #2#2#2#2#2#2
   #1#1#1#1#1#1#1
```

Now, in addition to three necessary behaviors, I need to introduce you to three principles that are an integral part in your success. As I explain them, the importance of each principle will make good sense, the light will go on, and you will have that "aha" moment. You'll never forget, and that's part of the plan.

Overcoming obesity is no trick, no sleight of hand, and no magic pill that instantly or effortlessly gives you what you want. These three powerful principles make an acronym, which makes it easy to remember and therefore easier to implement.

H: Hormones

A: Attitude

T: Timing

This is something that you cannot pull out of your hat, but when you understand and apply these three principles, it does make weight loss a whole lot easier!

H.A.T.–H IS FOR HORMONES

The fact that our bodies produce many different hormones that regulate more things than we will probably ever know is really no news flash. We hear the phrase "hormone imbalance" thrown around all the time, whether we know what that truly means or not.

But when dealing with appetite, hunger, and obesity, there are two key hormones that you must be familiar with. Those are:

Leptin: This hormone tells your body that you are *full.*
Grehlin: This hormone tells your body that you are *hungry.*

Imagine for a moment that you ate lunch, a good-sized lunch, and you are full. You are happy. Then suddenly something happens . . . and you are hungry again! What would you do? Naturally, you would eat more.

Or even worse, imagine that your body never tells you that you are full! Those pesky little appetite hormones can really be our undoing. Just a little off-kilter and—*BAM!*

Want to know what tilts your leptin and ghrelin hormones, thus sending you conflicting signals about your appetite and hunger? It pays to know, but it pays even more to apply that knowledge to your life.

The *International Journal of Obesity* reported on the research undertaken at the Metabolic Research Laboratory of the University Hospital of Navarra. The study was practical in that it explained both the power of the leptin and ghrelin hormones and showed how to manage the hormones. From a medical standpoint, that is great information, but from a personal perspective, that is life for my patients!

It doesn't take a rocket scientist to guess that when these two hormones are out of balance, losing weight is not only difficult, it is next to impossible. We can all take that much for granted.

> **DIET**
>
> MSG/artificial sweeteners mess up your hunger hormones.

The *ghrelin hormone* is what tells your body that you are hungry, and as expected, it kicks in right before your next meal. They found in the study that ghrelin levels decrease for about three hours after a meal, and then begin to increase again. During those three hours, you aren't very hungry. Yes, you just ate, but your ghrelin levels are low. Keep that in mind.

This is where things begin to get interesting, though it makes perfect sense. Generally speaking, the lower our levels of ghrelin, the less body fat we usually have. This is super important because ghrelin is constantly working to form abdominal fat near the liver, and that of course increases our risks of developing type 2 diabetes.

Quite clearly, we are fighting the gremlin ghrelin. It is a hormone we must keep in check. We want that hormone at low levels all the time.

The *leptin hormone*, on the other hand, tells your body that you are full. Your appetite, hunger, metabolism, and behavior are naturally affected by your leptin levels.

You are probably thinking, "Okay, then how can I increase my leptin levels so that my body knows it's full?"

That is indeed the right question to ask, but here is where most of us are getting off track. The study found that the foods we eat either (A) block our leptin levels, or (B) increase our leptin levels.

Obviously, to (A) block the leptin levels is not good, as that would mean the trigger of "stop eating, you are full" would never be pulled.

It is the second effect of leptin that is affecting us most.

"But how can part (B) of increased leptin levels be bad?" you may be wondering. "I thought you just said that higher leptin levels told my body that it was full."

Here is the problem. When the foods we eat are the wrong foods, our body does the reverse and produces *too much* leptin, so much so that our bodies become "leptin resistant," very similar to insulin-resistant people who have type 2 diabetes. In fact, most diabetics are also leptin resistant.

What foods are messing us up?

Well, in our society we are pretty much consuming the exact opposite of what we should be eating! The study found that leptin resistance happens when we eat low-nutrient foods like sodas, refined flours, candy, or any form of sugar.

These wrong foods block the leptin hormone so we don't feel

> **HEALTH**
>
> Foods that may be inflammatory: eat on occasion and with moderation.

full or they dump excessive leptin hormones into our blood stream so that we couldn't feel full even if we tried!

The good news is that leptin levels are in direct proportion to our body weight, which means that as we lose weight, our body will eventually become more sensitive to leptin. With less leptin being blocked and with less leptin resistance, you will eventually have less hunger and be able to control your appetite.

Now for the good part! Let's get practical and discuss real ways to control these ghrelin and leptin hormones. Again, the answer is through the food you eat and through the lifestyle that you choose to create. This will help:

- *Avoid MSG*: MSG messes with your leptin hormone, so you eat more and get hungrier sooner. MSG is typically in fast foods, processed foods, and more. (See www.msgtruth.org/avoid.htm for a comprehensive list of common foods with MSG.)
- *Avoid or minimize fructose*: Fructose prevents leptin and insulin from elevating to normal levels after a meal, which then increases your ghrelin and triglyceride levels, and you eat more. Fructose is in fruit juices and soft drinks.
- *Avoid low-calorie (1000 calories or less a day) diets*: Eating food helps balance hormones that trigger uncontrollable hunger and weight gain.
- *Eat every four hours*: Ghrelin is produced and secreted on a four-hour cycle. To keep ghrelin low, eat on schedule every three to four hours. Leptin levels are decreased after fasting 24 to 72 hours.
- *Eat high fiber foods*: Ghrelin levels remain high until food stretches the wall of your stomach, making you feel full.

High-volume, low-calorie, nutrient-dense foods reduce ghrelin and increase leptin levels long before you have eaten too much. Salads are good.

- *Get at least seven hours of sleep a night*: Less sleep means higher ghrelin levels, lower leptin levels, greater hunger, and higher body weight.
- *Eat proteins at every meal*: Protein takes longer to digest and lowers your ghrelin levels.
- *Reduce stress*: Take short walks, meditate, take a bath, do yoga, listen to soothing music.
- *Increase omega-3 fats*: This both boosts leptin and helps knock out leptin resistance. Grass-fed meats, walnuts, salmon, anchovies, sardines, trout, chia seeds, flax seeds, summer squash, and kale are good.
- *Heal your gut*: This helps with appetite issues.

Clearly, this is a vicious cycle, one that must be broken as quickly as possible! The modified Mediterranean Diet is a great answer because it helps to balance these two important appetite hormones.

H.A.T.–A IS FOR ATTITUDE

Our own attitude plays a part in weight loss. I have said for years that a positive mental attitude is one of the greatest keys to any successful endeavor. Sadly, I have witnessed the power of "stinkin' thinkin'" do untold damage in people's lives, especially when it comes to weight loss.

Most obese people (and yo-yo dieters) have a negative attitude that clouds their thinking. Sometimes the negative words seep out and I will hear things like:

"My whole family is fat, so I have the genes to be fat." That is not true! Yes, genetics may load the gun, but your environment and/or your food and lifestyle choices pull the trigger. Replace the lie with, "I have inherited genes that will help me lose weight." That *is* true.

"I've always been fat and I'll always be fat." That is not true either. Replace that lie with, "I will make healthy dietary choices and will exercise regularly and weight will drop off." That is also true.

"I have a slow metabolism" or *"I can't give up my comfort foods."* Both of these are lies. Get a vision of yourself thin and able to wear that pair of jeans you like. Say, "I see myself wearing those jeans." If you can envision it, you can achieve it. And you do have a metabolism that works fine.

We are body, mind, and spirit, and it's also important to address the spiritual components of weight loss. These are truths that I believe, and that you should as well:

- "I can do all things through Christ who strengthens me" (Philippians 4:13).
- "With God, all things are possible" (Matthew 19:26b).

You must remove the word "can't" from your vocabulary, from your conscious and subconscious vocabulary, and reprogram yourself with an I-will-not-be-denied attitude. This can-do thinking will take you where you want to go!

Any time a lie (negative words) flits across your mind, grab it by the heels and throw it down. Then stomp on it by speaking the truth. If a variation of "I'm so fat and ugly" comes zipping by, slap it down, then squish it with something like, "I accept myself, I forgive myself, and I love myself!"

Always confess the positive and reframe the negative. Come up with your own positive affirmations, and say them every morning and every night. If you hate your body, you attract more bad feelings and more weight gain, so you know that is a dead-end street. Reprogram yourself with can-do thinking.

Here are several can-do confessions:

- I forgive myself for gaining weight; I accept myself and forgive myself.
- I can lose weight and I am losing weight every week.
- I commit now to removing all junk foods, sugary foods, and tempting foods from my house.
- I commit now to eating three meals a day and a healthy mid-afternoon snack.
- I commit to eating breakfast like a king, lunch like a prince, and dinner like a pauper.
- I commit to practicing portion control.
- I commit now to practicing mindful eating.
- I give my body what it needs and not what it craves.
- I commit now to a regular physical activity program.
- I see myself weighing _____.

We all need to be grateful for the body we have, even if you are presently obese or overweight. Accept yourself, forgive yourself, and love yourself daily, and you will eventually change your auto-pilot to weight loss.

You have thousands of thoughts every day, and it's impossible to tune in to all of them. You can, however, tune in to your feelings.

When you are feeling down or blue, you are thinking negative thoughts. Conversely, when you are feeling great, you are thinking positive thoughts. Learn to tune in to your feelings, not your thoughts, so that you will be able to reframe the negative or stinkin' thinkin' into can-do thinking and positive confessions. The more you can practice gratitude and thanksgiving, the more positive thoughts you will have. When you practice gratitude, you automatically start smiling more, singing more, laughing more, playing more, and weight starts dropping off.

> **TRENDING**
>
> A waist measurement of 35" for women and 40" for men is usually associated with pre-diabetes.

On a practical note, you should:

- Drink 1–2 quarts of water daily, beginning as soon as you wake up.
- Exercise 15–30 minutes daily, with a good walk in the morning.
- Repeat your can-do confessions morning and night.
- Follow your eating plan.

A big part of a positive mental attitude is having a plan . . . we have one.

And knowing how to balance our hunger hormones . . . we know what that takes.

And knowing we are not alone . . . we know that.

And knowing what to do . . . we have that.

And we have a practical lifestyle diet that is proven to be effective . . . we have that with the modified Mediterranean Diet.

Now, it's time to get it done!

H.A.T.–T IS FOR TIMING

Not only is *what* we eat important, so is *when* we eat it. At the common-sense level, this is only logical. You have no doubt seen a race where people are handing out cups of water or energy bars as the runners pass. At that precise moment, those runners needed that intake of liquids or food. Yesterday's intake or last week's intake would of course mean nothing at that moment.

The timing is what is important. With weight loss, timing is incredibly important, as you will soon see.

The Tel Aviv University conducted a very interesting study (by Professor Daniela Jakubowicz and Dr. Julio Wainstein) that not only sheds light on the power of timing, it sheds pounds in a major way.[9]

For the study, they chose ninety-three obese women and randomly assigned them to eat the same foods (totaling 1400 calories) for twelve weeks. Half of the women ate at the same timing as we usually do, with a small breakfast (they were allowed 200 calories), medium lunch (500 calories), and big dinner (700 calories), while the other half had the exact opposite. This was the big shift in timing. They had their 1400 calories in reverse, with 700 calories for breakfast, 500 calories for lunch, and 200 calories at dinner.

BREAKFAST

The USDA reports that 44 percent of Americans eat breakfast every day, which means 56 percent are not eating breakfast at all. Our children do what we do.

Fast-forward twelve weeks and the statistics were staggering! The "big breakfast" group had lost, on average, 17.8 pounds each, not to mention 3 inches off their waistline! The "big dinner" group? They had lost just 7.3 pounds and only 1.4 inches at the waist.

The difference was *timing*.

As amazing as this was to see, all of these changes were on the outside. Remember, there is always something happening at the hormonal, metabolic, and biochemical levels. At this level, few people are aware of what is happening, but you need to be aware, for it will be mental and physical ammunition for your weight loss fight!

When they checked the "big breakfast" group, it was found that they had significantly lower levels of ghrelin (which you do want to be lower as it means a decreased appetite), which showed greater food satisfaction and was reflected in less of a desire to snack later in the day.

FOODS THAT USUALLY LEAD TO WEIGHT LOSS

1. Green tea
2. Leafy green vegetables
3. Wild salmon
4. Dark chocolate
5. Greek yogurt
6. Berries, lemons, limes, Granny Smith apples
7. Steel-cut oats

The "big dinner" group was not so lucky. They had higher levels of ghrelin, they were hungrier, and they wanted to snack more often.

What's more, the "big breakfast" group also had lower levels of insulin, glucose, and triglyceride (a type of fat in the body). On the health meter, that translates directly into a lower risk of diabetes, cardiovascular disease, hypertension, and high cholesterol. The "big dinner" group actually had increased levels of triglycerides, despite their weight loss.

If that wasn't enough, the "big breakfast" group did not have the normal high spikes of blood glucose levels that occur after a meal. It is these peaks in blood sugar levels that are considered dangerous, even more harmful than sustained high blood glucose levels, all of which leads to insulin resistance, pre-diabetes, or diabetes.

The study conclusively showed just how important timing is to weight loss. Within three months, the "big breakfast" group proved that fact by losing almost three times as much weight as the "big dinner" group in spite of the fact that they had the exact same number of calories each day.

> **THOUGHT**
>
> Most chronic diseases are choice diseases. We don't *catch* them; we *develop* them by consistently choosing the wrong foods.

Interestingly, in another Tel Aviv University study in 2012, study subjects added dessert to their breakfast, including cookies, cake, or chocolate. The study this time lasted thirty-two weeks, and the "big breakfast" group lost an average of forty pounds more than the group that ate a small breakfast, medium lunch, and large dinner but avoided cookies, chocolate, and cake.[10]

Sadly, the "big dinner" group gained their weight back.

YOUR NEXT WEIGHT-LOSS STEPS

If you are looking to lose weight, know that you hold in your hands the key you have been looking for. Not only will it unlock the door to weight loss, but it will unlock the door to a healthy lifestyle, and that is off-the-charts amazing! Years from now, you can look back with joy and satisfaction.

You will also be looking at diseases from the other side of the fence. Those thirty-five diseases that are directly related to obesity? You will most likely not even have to worry about them! How is that for a happy thought?

Now, it takes three weeks to create a habit, so don't be too hard on yourself if it takes some time for this to feel like the "new you." It also takes a few weeks for the weight to begin coming off.

You are changing history, right here and now. Your good food choices are going to make a huge impact in your life, in your wallet, and in the lives of those around you who love you dearly.

Don't let the statistics scare you anymore. I read recently from the *Journal of American Medical Association* that one in three Americans are obese, followed by the American Diabetes Association that states that one in three Americas have diabetes or are pre-diabetic (of that number, 90–95 percent are type 2 diabetic). The diabetes epidemic is following the obesity epidemic, but it's a train you don't have to ride.

Let those statistics motivate you to change your world. You can get off that train and chart your own course to freedom!

THE MODIFIED MEDITERRANEAN DIET'S
BIG BREAKFAST/SMALL DINNER PLAN

I put together a big breakfast/small dinner diet for my patients. It truly is working wonders and it meshes well with the modified Mediterranean Diet. If losing weight is your focus, I suggest that you shift from the modified Mediterranean Diet to the modified Mediterranean Diet's big breakfast/small dinner plan for at least twelve weeks. Continue for another twelve weeks if you want, then swap back to the modified Mediterranean Diet for a season. The modified Mediterranean Diet is a lifestyle that you can live with long term.

BREAKFAST (600–700 calories): Rotate daily.

Meal #1: Steel-cut oatmeal; you can add stevia, a handful of berries, a handful of walnuts or pecans if you want. Along with this, you can have a protein drink or smoothie with 8 ounces of almond or coconut milk, 1 teaspoon of coconut oil or almond butter for your good fats, one scoop of plant protein, and 1–2 tbsp. ground flaxseed for your fiber. May add ice or stevia to taste.

Meal #2: Eggs (3 whites and 1 yolk is best) or an omelet with onions, peppers, or any other vegetables; a little cheese or a few slices of avocado is okay. You can have 2 slices of gluten free toast (Canyon Bakery gluten-free bread is my favorite and is often found in the frozen section of a health food store.) with a little butter or a little almond butter.

Meal #3: Greek yogurt or low-fat cottage cheese with berries and stevia, and a protein drink or smoothie with almond or coconut milk, almond butter or coconut oil, a scoop of plant protein, and 1–2 tbsp. ground flaxseeds. May add ice or stevia to taste.

Meal #4: Gluten-free pancakes with berries (blueberries, blackberries, strawberries, or raspberries) sautéed in a small amount of butter or coconut oil (not syrup). May add 3–4 oz. of smoked wild salmon, 2 slices of turkey bacon, or a protein drink or smoothie as above.

Coffee: Okay, just no sugar or cream. You can use stevia to sweeten, and almond or coconut milk in place of cream. Tea is also okay, just no sugar; use stevia or truvia.

LUNCH: No bread, pasta, rice, or potatoes.

You can have all salads with all the vegetables you want, but don't add croutons. A little cheese is fine, but not every day (rotating every three to four days). Add 3 to 6 ounces of protein such as chicken, turkey, or fish (3–4 oz. for women, 3–6 oz. for men).

You can have ½–1 cup of beans, peas, or lentils in soups or have hummus as side dish.

Use your olive oil and vinegar (use 2–4 parts vinegar and 1 part olive oil) in a salad spritzer, and other condiments like lemon or lime, garlic, pepper, or one-calorie per spray salad spritzers by Wishbone on salads. No creamy dressings (i.e., ranch, blue cheese, etc.).

DINNER: No starches, and no beans, peas, or lentils.

You can have salad with all your vegetables, but no croutons. You can add 3 to 6 ounces of protein such as chicken, turkey, or fish. You can have non-cream based vegetable soups and all the green vegetables you desire, such as cabbage, broccoli, asparagus, green beans, etc.

SNACKS:

Raw nuts
Organic celery and carrot sticks
Guacamole or avocado
Lettuce wraps
Salsa is okay, but with no chips
Hot tea is okay with no sugar (use stevia or Truvia)

NOTES TO REMEMBER:

1. Make sure you eat dinner at around 6 or 7 p.m., and go to bed early, around 9 to 10 p.m., so you don't get late night cravings. This helps both control and rebalance your ghrelin and leptin hormones. Sleep deprivation usually increases appetite.
2. Drink 2 glasses of water as soon as you wake up. This is great for weight loss and getting rid of body toxins first thing in the morning.
3. Exercise thirty minutes a day, five days a week, and try to get your heart rate up to 120–130 beats per minute. A recumbent bike is recommended to keep pressure off your knees. Try a brisk walk in the morning before breakfast for burning belly fat.
4. Control your stress. That also affects your appetite hormones. Learn to let it go, forgive, and move on.

Does the Big Breakfast/Small Dinner diet work? Yes.

Will you lose weight? Yes.

In fact, I can promise you that if you'll stick to the diet, as thousands of other people have, you will reap the benefits, both in weight loss as well as in creating a healthy lifestyle that will serve you well for the rest of your life.

Jason came to see me. His expanding waistline of 42 inches told me he was pre-diabetic at the minimum, which he was. He had crossed from being overweight to being obese and he was sick of it. My warning that he was about to be sicker was fuel to his fire. He was motivated to take action.

> ## LIFESTYLE
>
> Eat breakfast like a king, lunch like a prince, and dinner like a pauper.

I explained the three behaviors (good food choices, good beverage choices, and physical activity). That made sense to him, but as I outlined the modified Mediterranean Diet and then the Big Breakfast/Medium Lunch/Small Dinner diet, I could see him start to squirm. He was fighting an internal struggle, one that involved giving up his daily comfort foods.

The fact that he could enjoy smaller portions of his comfort foods, on occasion, did help, but when I began to list the thirty-five diseases that obesity was directly connected to, not to mention the financial costs that would come from being obese, something seemed to snap inside of him. His light came on—I could almost hear it!

He was on board from that moment forward. He stuck to the diet and followed my instructions, which balanced his hunger hormones and improved his attitude. He managed his meal timing and went on walks regularly with his wife. Within weeks, he was losing weight. Within months, he wasn't even pre-diabetic.

When I asked what his internal motivation was, which I know is our strongest possible motivator, he said, "I'm not done living yet. I have too many things I want to do with my loved ones. I also don't want to spend all my hard-earned retirement income on medical bills."

We both chuckled, but it was true. The light that turned on with his "aha" moment meant a bright future ahead for Jason and his family.

SECTION TWO

Applying the Answers

CHAPTER SIX

℞

YOUR JOURNEY

Chapter Six marks the beginning of Section Two, where you can apply the answers to your life and treat the specific disease that torments you. Armed with the modified Mediterranean Diet, you can combat the horrifying national statistics of heart disease. Learn how to effectively treat heart disease and a host of other heart-related ailments with your food.

Don Colbert, MD

BEAT CARDIOVASCULAR DISEASES

with the Modified Mediterranean Diet

MANY YEARS AGO, Jim had a heart attack. With about a 75 percent blockage in his left coronary artery, the doctors put him on medicines right away. Jim then came to see me. After a thorough review, we took action.

I put him on the Mediterranean Diet (this was before we modified it) and started him on a nutritional program, along with antioxidants, which are low with most people who have heart disease. I also identified and modified with diet and nutritional supplements all of his cardiovascular risk factors.

More than ten years went by. He was on the Mediterranean Diet for much of the time, but was flexible, occasionally having a bowl of ice cream or some other treat. For the most part he followed the system, and the results spoke for themselves. He lost a lot of belly fat and his blood pressure, cholesterol, triglycerides, C-reactive protein (CRP), and sugar levels were all under control.

Then one day he started experiencing chest pains again! He went back to his same cardiologist and they ran several tests, including a repeat heart cath. When the doctor walked into the room, he was shaking his head. "This is amazing," he said. "I've been practicing for decades and I have never seen anything like this. Here is a picture of your left coronary artery ten or so years ago when it was 75 percent blocked."

Jim looked at the pictures. The blockage was very evident.

"But now," the doctor went on, placing a new image on the table, "ten years later, you have only a 20 percent blockage. I've never seen that before. What have you been doing?"

The plaque was reversing itself! When Jim told me his story, I knew we were on target for our patients, and this was years ago when it was the straight unmodified Mediterranean Diet. Now it's even better!

Oh, and the chest pains he was experiencing? It turned out to be acid reflux, something we fixed in no time.

HEART DISEASE IS KILLING US!

For years now, heart disease has been the number one killer of those in the United States—and that is true for both men and women.[11] The CDC reports that there are other "medical conditions and lifestyle choices" that also play a part in putting people at a higher risk for heart disease, including:

- Hypertension
- Diabetes
- Overweight and obesity
- Poor diet
- Physical inactivity
- Excessive alcohol use
- Smoking history
- High cholesterol

That is certainly not a news flash. And with the steadily increasing number of people with diabetes and obesity, the number of deaths from heart disease is only going to increase.

If that isn't a dark enough picture, according to the Mayo Clinic, those with heart disease can expect to live with these complications:

- *Heart failure*: The heart can't pump enough blood to meet the body's needs.
- *Heart attack*: A blood clot blocks the blood flow through a blood vessel that feeds the heart, causing a heart attack, possibly damaging or destroying a part of the heart muscle.
- *Stroke*: The risk factors that lead to cardiovascular disease also can lead to an ischemic stroke (when arteries to the brain are narrowed or blocked, and too little blood reaches the brain). The brain tissue begins to die within just a few minutes of a stroke.
- *Aneurysm*: This is a bulge in the wall of the artery. If an aneurysm bursts, the patient may face life-threatening internal bleeding.
- *Peripheral artery disease*: The extremities (usually the legs) don't receive enough blood flow, causing leg pain when walking.
- *Sudden cardiac arrest*: The sudden, unexpected loss of heart function, breathing, and consciousness. If not treated immediately, it is fatal.

According to the Heart Foundation, someone in the United States has a heart attack every thirty-four seconds, and every sixty seconds, one of those heart attack victims dies. Those numbers are hard to fathom.

I don't know your story or your situation, but if you are suffering from heart disease in any way, shape, or form, let's work together to get you back on solid ground. You cannot be one of these statistics!

One effective motivator that is powerful enough to cause people to take action (I have seen this to be true countless times) is clarifying your "why" for getting healthy. Why do you want to get your health back? Why do you want to beat heart disease?

CRAVINGS

Those with heart disease, artery blockage, and obesity typically crave: *deep fried foods*.

Work on that, refine it until it's a burning white-hot passion that drives you to do whatever it takes to be healthy. Let it propel you to where you want to go, which is a healthy lifestyle that gives you the life and freedom that you want!

IT'S ALL HEART RELATED

Everything we are talking about for heart disease also holds true for all things heart related, such as high blood pressure, high cholesterol, and high triglycerides. Each of these can usually be effectively treated, and usually controlled, and sometimes reversed by following the modified Mediterranean Diet.

According to the CDC, seventy million Americans have high blood pressure, and even more have high cholesterol! That's a *third* of the country's adults.

Quite expectedly, a third of the nation also has high triglycerides. These triglycerides are fatty particles found in your blood, along with LDL cholesterol (the bad cholesterol) and HDL (the good cholesterol).

Looking at cholesterol for a second, you want to lower your LDL cholesterol to less than 100 and raise your HDL over 55. By losing weight (especially the belly fat), cutting wheat, corn, and sugar from your diet, avoiding trans fats, and pulling the plug on fried foods, you will be well on your way to doing just that. Get on the modified Mediterranean Diet with some relevant supplements, and your LDL and HDL numbers will start to come in line.

That's treating the whole person and the root cause, and laying the groundwork for a healthy person. That is also the way it should be.

FOODS THAT USUALLY RAISE BLOOD PRESSURE

- Table salt, baking soda, baking powder
- Sauces (teriyaki, soy), salad dressings
- Cured meat (beef jerky), cured fish
- Cheese
- Pickles and canned vegetables
- Instant soups
- Roasted and salted nuts and seeds, pretzels, chips

However, most doctors see only the red flashing light that blinks "lower cholesterol, lower cholesterol," and since that is often their only goal, they prescribe statin drugs (i.e., Lipitor, Lescol, Crestor, and Zocor, to name only a few) to everyone. These medications were designed to save our lives, and they may do just that . . . but they were not designed to treat our symptoms while we continue to ignore the root cause of the sickness.

The prolonged use of these drugs, however, is producing bad side effects. I am not the only doctor to see these drugs stress and inflame the liver, decrease energy and sex hormones, lower coenzyme Q10 levels, affect the mind, potentially lead to dementia and Alzheimer's, and more.

Forbes magazine reported back in 2013 that over 400,000 deaths each year are from preventable medical errors, and that number includes prescriptions that obviously did more harm than good.[12] This death-by-doctor error ranks as the number three killer, behind heart disease (number one) and cancer (number two).

Though I hold doctors and the big pharmacy companies responsible for the massive prescriptions of statin drugs and the ensuing effects, it is really the individual taking the pill who is ultimately responsible.

I told one patient, "It's your life. You get to choose what goes in your mouth."

Tough as that is to say, she smiled and replied, "I really can't argue with that."

Recently, I had a middle-aged man come into my office who was taking four medications for his high blood pressure. It was necessary at the time, but he knew he didn't want to stay on the medications. He was also suffering from fatigue, erectile dysfunction, and dizziness, which were side effects of his blood pressure medications.

He started on the modified Mediterranean Diet, eliminating all wheat and corn, and began exercising. The results were not instant, but within three months, he was off his first blood pressure drug. He lost weight, his waist decreased by three

FOODS THAT USUALLY LOWER BLOOD PRESSURE

- Pomegranates
- Olive leaf, olive oil
- Dark chocolate
- Garlic
- Asparagus, kale, spinach
- Celery
- Beets

inches, and his blood pressure dropped 20 points. By the end of the sixth month, he was off another drug. Going from four to two is good, and his fatigue, erectile dysfunction, and dizziness were gone! In time, he may be able to come off more medications, but he is on his way, and he was excited about getting his health back.

I have literally had hundreds of people reverse their high blood pressure, high cholesterol, and high triglycerides by following the modified Mediterranean Diet. One of the first things that happens is that they usually start to burn off their belly fat, and that alone often cuts down one or more blood pressure medications!

> ### EAT MORE
>
> Natural ways to increase nitric oxide levels include: beets, pine bark extract, grape seed extract, pomegranate, and citrulline and arginine supplements.

If you are suffering from heart disease or dealing with high blood pressure, high cholesterol, or high triglycerides, then the time is now to get started on your modified Mediterranean Diet.

THE MODIFIED MEDITERRANEAN DIET FOR HEART DISEASE

Below is the same foundational modified Mediterranean Diet, except in several places you will see that it is altered slightly to best decrease inflammation for heart disease, high blood pressure, high cholesterol, and high triglycerides.

Level #1: fruits, vegetables, nuts, beans, and other legumes. Salads consist of dark green leafy lettuce, fresh vine-ripened tomatoes, broccoli, spinach, peppers, onions, and cucumbers. Serve vegetables in salads, as appetizers, or as a main or side dish. Fruits are usually a dessert or snack. Use nuts as toppings to add flavor and texture. The beans and legumes are usually in soups, added to salads, used as dips (i.e., hummus), or as a main dish.

Suggestions: Start with a large salad with lunch and dinner (no croutons). Eat vegetables three servings a day and more if able. Eat raw, steam, stir-fry, or cook under low heat with olive oil, macadamia nut oil, or coconut oil. Eat fruits two or more servings a day (blueberries, blackberries, strawberries, raspberries, lemons, limes, or any other types of fruit—but avoid fruit juice).

Suggestions: Eat ½ to 2 cups daily of beans, bean soups, peas, lentils, legumes, and hummus, preferably before meals.

Level #2: steel-cut oats and quinoa, millet or millet bread, brown rice, brown rice pasta, brown rice bread, and sweet potatoes.

Altered: Eliminate wheat, corn, and white rice completely from your diet. When your cardiovascular disease is controlled, you can rotate sprouted bread (Ezekiel 4:9 bread) or fermented bread (sourdough) and organic non-processed corn every four days or less often and with moderation.

Level #3: olive oil used instead of other oils, margarine, etc. Not only for cooking, it is commonly mixed with balsamic vinegar as a salad dressing. It's best to avoid butter.

Altered: Limit salt in your diet to 1.5 grams (1,500 milligrams) a day.

Altered: Eliminate all fried foods completely from your diet.

Suggestions: Consume 2 to 4 tablespoons of extra-virgin olive oil daily, with cooking and on salads (with balsamic vinegar or any other type of vinegar).

Suggestions: Eat one handful of raw nuts (almonds, hazelnuts, pecans, cashews, walnuts, macadamia) daily.

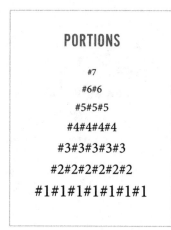

PORTIONS

#7
#6#6
#5#5#5
#4#4#4#4
#3#3#3#3#3
#2#2#2#2#2#2
#1#1#1#1#1#1#1

Level #4: cheese and yogurt, in small amounts. Freshly grated Parmesan on pasta or a little feta cheese on a salad is common. Yogurt (about a cup) is how milk is usually eaten, and it is low fat or nonfat, served with fresh fruit added. Yogurt is also used in salad dressing (i.e., mixed with dill, garlic, onion, and cucumbers). Rotate dairy every four days.

Altered: May use low-fat yogurt or unsweetened low-fat cottage cheese, and add your own fruit, rotating the dairy every four days. (Caution: cottage cheese has a moderate amount of sodium.)

Level #5: fish (low mercury fish, see Appendix C), eaten more than other meats, in about 4- to 6-ounce portions several times a week.

Level #6: chicken, turkey, and eggs. Chicken in 3- to 6-ounce portions a few times a week is common. The meat is usually skinless and added to soups, stews, and other dishes loaded with vegetables.

Only 1 to 2 egg yolks per week. I recommend 1 egg yolk with 3 egg whites once/twice a week.

Suggestions: If you grill, thinly slice meat and marinate in red wine, juice (pomegranate, cherry), or curry sauce. Remove any char from meat.

Level #7: 3 to 6 ounces of red meat, in the form of beef, veal, pork, sheep, lamb, and goat, is eaten once or twice a week at most. It is usually served as a topping to a vegetable, pasta, or rice dish.

Suggestions: Rotate vegetables and meats every 4 days (do not eat the same foods every day). For example, day 1 eat chicken and then day 2 turkey and day 3 salmon and so on.

FOODS THAT TYPICALLY RAISE CHOLESTEROL

- Fried foods
- Wheat, bread, bagels, white pasta, pretzels
- Processed corn (tortillas, corn chips, corn flour)
- Trans fats (margarine, cake icing, donuts, Bisquick Original)
- Ice cream, non-dairy creamer, cheese, butter, whole milk
- Ground beef, bacon, sausage, hot dogs, saturated fats (marbled and fatty meats)
- Processed foods (pastries, cookies, microwave popcorn)

IT COMES BACK TO INFLAMMATION

Inflammation is the root cause for heart disease and the related high blood pressure, high cholesterol, and high triglycerides.

As we discussed earlier, acute inflammation is the good side of inflammation, such as the red, painful swelling around a splinter. It's part of the healing and if treated correctly, it's very short lived.

With chronic inflammation, the body creates cytokines, little proteins that are both inflammatory and "sticky." This constricts the blood vessels, which raises your blood pressure and sets the stage for a blood clot. The perfect recipe for a heart attack or stroke, wouldn't you say?

The source of the inflammation, as you know, is most commonly the food we eat . . . and the modified Mediterranean Diet effectively decreases the "stickiness" caused by acute inflammation, and that directly lowers your blood pressure and reduces your risks of a heart attack.

> **LIFESTYLE**
>
> Most people with heart issues also have obesity to deal with.

Even the unmodified Mediterranean Diet is a huge step in the right direction. The *New York Times* reported several years ago that "about 30 percent of heart attacks, strokes, and deaths from heart disease can be prevented in people at high risk if they switch to a Mediterranean Diet rich in olive oil, nuts, beans, fish, fruits and vegetables, and even drink wine with meals, a large and rigorous new study has found."

Remember the fellow at the start of this chapter? He had 75 percent blockage in his left coronary artery, but after being on the Mediterranean Diet (and even loosely at that), his body cleared itself of the plaque down to only a 20 percent blockage. Out went the food that was causing the inflammation and out went the results of that inflammation.

When I'm working with a patient who suffers from high blood pressure, I get them off corn and wheat right away, and decrease their salt dramatically. They had better watch out! It's usually a fast and big drop in their numbers! I warn them that they may come down fast, so if they are taking medications and are starting the modified Mediterranean Diet at the same time, they need to monitor their blood pressure regularly. Typically, in three months they are usually able to reduce the amount they take of one of their medications—or eliminate it completely! Also, as one loses belly fat, the blood pressure usually drops accordingly.

I have found that many patients with high blood pressure also suffer from sleep apnea. Weight loss often takes care of it.

If you want to get on the modified Mediterranean Diet for both weight loss and heart disease issues, the answer is simple: go back and forth. If, for example, your blood pressure is not coming down, switch over to the modified Mediterranean Diet's Big Breakfast/ Small Dinner plan for weight loss to get the belly fat off, and then switch back after your blood pressure is down.

Many times, the modified Mediterranean Diet is sufficient by itself to reach the desired health goals. The beauty of having the modified Mediterranean Diet as the foundation, because it is such a healthy long-term lifestyle, is that you are free to slide back and forth as needed. And if you don't have ailments, the modified Mediterranean Diet is both a great lifestyle and the best preventive

FOODS THAT USUALLY LOWER CHOLESTEROL

- Seeds (flax, chia, salba, psyllium)
- Soluble fiber (beans, peas, legumes, lentils)
- Wild salmon, wild sardines
- Steel-cut oats
- Avocado, olive oil
- Walnuts, almonds, cashews
- Garlic

medicine around! Once your health condition is controlled, you can rotate an avoidance food every four days in a limited amount.

Being diagnosed with heart disease or being prescribed heart medications that are "for the rest of your life" are very tough burdens to bear. Fear is often an ever-present companion . . . at least it was with me.

Now, you can look forward to the future with the modified Mediterranean Diet! That may sound like pure fiction to some, but for many, it is no longer just a hope . . . it's a proven fact.

Clive came into my office with high blood pressure, high cholesterol, type 2 diabetes, and elevated PSA, and he was on medications

> ### PRESSURE RISING
>
> These negative emotions contribute to high blood pressure:
>
> - anger
> - hostility
> - resentment
> - frustration,
> - irritability

for all these conditions. I put him on the best anti-inflammatory diet in the world (the modified Mediterranean Diet), with specific instructions to avoid wheat, corn, sugar, fried food, and trans fats. We lowered his salt intake and got him walking briskly thirty minutes a day. I added in a few supplements, such as the inexpensive vitamin D.

Is that doable? It certainly is, but when it comes to your health, it's more than doable!

Three short months later, Clive had dropped thirty pounds. And here are the results of his taking action:

- Blood pressure: normal
- Blood sugar levels: normal

- Cholesterol levels: normal
- PSA levels: normal

I don't think he is too worried about heart disease at this point, nor is he worried about the damaging effects of the medications . . . because he isn't taking any of them any longer!

CHAPTER SEVEN

R/

YOUR JOURNEY

Chapter Seven is all about arthritis, from rheumatoid to osteoarthritis, and the complications and remedies that you might be facing. If you suffer from arthritis, you will benefit from knowing how to find answers to your questions. Control what inflames you, jump on the modified Mediterranean Diet, and you'll be well on your way to health again!

Don Colbert, MD

BEAT ARTHRITIS AND AUTOIMMUNE DISEASE
with the Modified Mediterranean Diet

SUSAN HAD DEVELOPED severe rheumatoid arthritis, already showing signs of deformities in her fingers. It looked like a dark future ahead since Susan was only in her early twenties.

Her rheumatologist had prescribed a list of medications, but she didn't want the side effects. When she came to me, I put her on the anti-inflammatory modified Mediterranean Diet. We cut out dairy, gluten, night shades (peppers, tomatoes, potatoes, paprika, eggplant), corn, and fried foods. I put her on a few anti-inflammatory supplements as well, such as krill oil, curcumin, and a supplement that boosts glutathione (an antioxidant and anti-inflammatory).

After six months, we started rotating back in the foods that typically cause inflammation for arthritis patients and she only ate small amounts of those foods every four days. Her inflammation was controlled with diet and supplements, and though her deformities (in her fingers) did not disappear, the deformities did not worsen any more.

With her life back to a new "normal" of controlled rheumatoid arthritis, she moved on. She got married, had two children, and the last time I heard from her, she was doing great. She is not on any of the medications that her rheumatologist originally put her on, and it has been several years since her initial diagnosis.

Looking back, if we had caught it earlier, we probably could have done even more. With some patients, if the rheumatoid arthritis is recently diagnosed and the inflammatory foods identified and eliminated, the effects of the anti-inflammatory diet may help the body revert back to what it was before, so they no longer test positive for the disease at all. I've seen that happen many times.

FOODS THAT USUALLY FUEL AUTOIMMUNE DISEASE

- Gluten (wheat, barley, rye)
- Gluten-free grains (corn)
- Nightshades (tomato, potato, paprika, peppers, eggplant)
- Sugar
- All genetically modified foods (GMOs)—soy, canola oil, cottonseed oil, beet sugar, papaya
- Trans fats, fried foods
- Polyunsaturated fats

A PAIN IN THE NECK!

According to the CDC, about 23 percent of the US population (over eighteen and not institutionalized) suffers from arthritis. The number is increasing as the population ages and becomes increasingly obese. Osteoarthritis is the most common form of arthritis, which usually affects the fingers, knees, neck, back, and hips. It is, quite simply, a degenerative joint disease.

Rheumatoid arthritis, on the other hand, is an autoimmune disorder that also causes joint pain, but is the result of cartilage and bone eroding away. It also can affect different organs in the body. The CDC reports that only about 1 percent of the population has rheumatoid arthritis and that the causes are unknown (and there is no known cure).

But osteoarthritis and rheumatoid arthritis, the two most common forms of arthritis, are more than just a pain in the neck. They are both associated with inflammation in the joints. With rheumatoid arthritis, we are talking about:

- Destroyed cartilage and bone
- Deformed bones
- Fused joints
- Increased risk for anemia (low red blood cell levels that bring about fatigue, weakness, dizziness)
- Rheumatoid lung (fluid in the lungs, scarring, lumps, high blood pressure in the lungs)
- Increased risks for heart disease
- Inability to do daily tasks
- Loss of job

With arthritis, the complications include:

- Inability to do daily tasks
- Pain and swelling in the joints
- Cannot walk comfortably or sit straight
- Twisted joints
- Deformation
- Loss of appetite
- Difficulty sleeping
- Depression[13]

It usually begins with joint pain, followed by redness, stiffness, and swelling (signs of acute inflammation). If the acute inflammation is not addressed, it leads to chronic inflammation, which leads to chronic pain, and if you ignore the pain, deformity usually follows.

Are you experiencing joint pain?

Don't ignore it. Your body has multiple warning systems in place, and the pain is usually a sign that inflammation is present. Identify the inflammatory foods and triggers and then eliminate those foods. In other words, fix it; don't cover it up or pretend it doesn't exist.

Imagine if the engine light comes on in your car. The little red "check the engine" light is flashing on your dashboard . . . are you going to ignore that light?

I used to park my car under my outdoor portico. I would pull my car around on the side of the house. It was a great spot, shaded and ready for quick access for work. One morning, I started the engine and heard the weirdest clicking and grinding sounds, but the car started up. The "check the engine" light popped on. I figured it was just a glitch, something out of balance that needed to be tweaked at 25,000 miles, which it had just reached. It was, after all, a new car. No big deal.

However, a few weeks later, that obnoxious "check the engine" light was still on and the clicking/grinding sound was getting worse, so I figured I would schedule my 25,000 mile tune-up and have him flip a switch or jiggle something. No doubt it would be fast.

I wasn't seated long when the mechanic came into the waiting area and said, "You need to see this, because if we didn't show you, you would think we were lying to you." He took me out into the bay where my car was hoisted up on a lift above our heads and he showed me numerous engine wires that were shredded. "You had a rat that got in under your hood and it chewed up your wires," he explained. "We need to basically replace all of these damaged wires."

My engine light was only trying to help me, and I had disregarded it for weeks. I was lucky I didn't break down beside the road or have something else break as a result.

Ignoring the problem would not have made it go away. I have heard about some people who actually pulled out the fuse for the blinking engine light. That is not very smart!

As for your body, figuratively speaking, you come equipped with warning lights that register pain. If you ignore the blinking "pain, pain, pain" red light, the pain will not go away. It's going to get worse and the warning light is usually inflammation triggering the pain.

When you do go to the doctor, standard protocol is to treat your symptoms. That's what we doctors are taught to do. Maybe they will help you mask it with drugs or pain medication so that you never need to address the real issue, but is that not similar to pulling the fuse?

Over time, it's only going to get worse . . . and you can't pull all the fuses out.

With my psoriasis, my primary irritant and source of inflammation was the gluten (eaten daily, at every meal) and peppers (eaten almost daily, in good-size portions). My small intestine was inflamed and unable to heal.

Had there been a pill to take away the itch and rash, or to even decrease the symptoms by the slightest of margins, I would have done it in a heartbeat. All the while, I would have gone on eating the very foods that were causing me problems.

The foods we eat usually either trigger diseases or add fuel to the fire. Either way, until we get to the source of the problem and truly fix it, we are most likely going to see more and more symptoms pop up. It is inevitable.

FOODS THAT USUALLY RELIEVE AUTOIMMUNE DISEASE

- Berries (blueberries, blackberries, raspberries, strawberries)
- Broccoli, cabbage, brussels sprouts
- Flaxseeds, salba seeds, chia seeds
- Healthy fats (olive oil, avocados)
- Wild salmon, wild sardines
- Almonds, walnuts, macadamia nuts
- Kale, spinach

INFLAMMATION IS A WARNING

Inflammation is another one of your body's warning lights that you should not ignore.

Several years ago, my wife, Mary, began experiencing pain in her right index finger. It really hurt, like she had sprained it or pulled it. Over time, the pain would lessen, but it would come back with a vengeance every so often.

She had no idea what was causing it, so she learned to live with it. Not much you can do about a painful, inflamed finger anyway . . . inflammation?

I had been studying the many links between food, inflammation, pain, and diseases. Could her one finger on one hand be a warning light, a sign that a certain food was causing pain and inflammation?

The next time it happened, I asked her, "What did you eat in the last twenty-four hours?"

BEAT ARTHRITIS AND AUTOIMMUNE DISEASE

"It's not the food," she replied, but she humored me, listing all that she had eaten in the last two days.

"I think it's the fried food you ate," I added. "So the next time you eat something fried, see how your finger is the following day."

Months later, her index finger was throbbing. It hurt worse than normal. The night before, we were together in a restaurant and she had eaten one of her favorite hors d'oeuvres: potato skins. She thought they were baked, but I asked and found that the potato skins were deep fried.

Since then, Mary has cut way back on all fried foods, and if she eats any, she eats just a little. The result? She has not experienced that throbbing, severe pain in her index finger ever since.

It wasn't the food itself (i.e., the potato skins) that was causing Mary trouble; it was the oils that her food was cooked in.

I have found polyunsaturated fats, such as corn oil, cotton seed oil, safflower oil, sunflower oil, and soybean oil, to be a major trigger for inflammation of the joints. A little bit is okay, but a lot is bad for you, especially if it is deep fried.

> **CRAVINGS**
>
> Those with osteo-arthritis typically crave: *dairy, fried foods, red meat, and nightshades.*

Unfortunately, these same oils are in most sauces, salad dressings, gravies, and cream-based products. Most fast food restaurants use these oils because they are good for cooking and they are cheap. The drawback is that the oils are also extremely inflammatory. If you frequently eat fast food, you are asking for pain in your joints.

With osteoarthritis, there is almost always a food that is causing the flare-up. Your job is to find that "thorn" and remove it. When you do, the pain will usually subside, the inflammation will diminish, and the joints will usually improve. Trouble comes when doctors give you an anti-inflammatory drug that enables you to keep eating the very foods that triggered the inflammation in the first place.

If you think you are sensitive to a specific food, you can perform your own food elimination test. As it relates to arthritis, eliminate processed meats (bacon, salami, pepperoni, sausage), corn, soy, wheat, pork, sugar, egg yolks, beef, shellfish, milk and dairy products, omega-6 fats or polyunsaturated fats (sunflower, safflower, corn, cottonseed, and soybean oil), nightshade plants (tomatoes, eggplant, potatoes, paprika, and peppers—bell, jalapeno, and cayenne), and fried foods from your diet.

Completely quit eating those foods for two to four weeks. Then for a week, eat one of the foods you eliminated. If you do not get any pain, redness, warmth, or swelling, then continue eating it. If you do get those symptoms, then you should stop eating that food for at least six months and after that only eat a small amount every four days or greater. Now many arthritis patients are sensitive to all the above inflammatory foods associated with arthritis.

> **HEALTH**
>
> Tart cherries usually relieve osteoarthritis pain.

Deformity may eventually come to our joints if we continue to ignore the warning signs. With all the pain and inflammation, I've found that the source of the problem almost always comes back to the food.

With osteoarthritis patients (and type 2 diabetic patients), we typically have a 90 percent improvement rate if the disease is caught in time and it's mainly their diet that we adjust. I've found the most common foods that cause the greatest inflammation to joints, for both men and women, are:

#1: Dairy (cheese, milk, ice cream, yogurt, sour cream)
#2: Fried food
#3: Red meat/pork/processed meats/shellfish
#4: Nightshades (tomatoes, potatoes, peppers, paprika, eggplant)
#5: Polyunsaturated fats (corn oil, cottonseed oil, sunflower oil, safflower oil)
#6: Trans fats (margarine, shortening, etc.)
#7: Corn
#8: Wheat

Could you go without these foods for a season, or forever, if it meant no longer having to worry about arthritis? Of course you could.

Soon after Mary and I were married, I noticed that her knees would pop and creak when she went up and down the stairs. "It's normal," she would say, but popping and creaking knees are not normal, much less for a young person. Usually it's a sign that your body is dehydrated in some way.

Depending on age and gender, we are made up of about 60–70 percent water, but our brain cells are about 85 percent water. Within our bodies, there are certain fluid levels that cannot go low. Your spinal fluid level is very important, as is your blood. But your synovial fluid that bathes the joints, the fluid that inflates the discs (those discs are 90 percent water), and digestive fluids are not as important as your spinal fluid or blood.

Sounds like a car again, doesn't it? You admittedly won't get far without gas, but if you run out of oil, you'll destroy your engine. But you can go a really long way without wiper fluid.

Here is what is interesting: Your body sacrifices certain fluids to keep the other fluids at the proper level. It will actually pull water from one place (i.e., your joints and discs) to hydrate another place (i.e., your spinal fluid). The lower priority reservoirs will be lowered in an effort to keep the higher priority reservoirs at maximum capacity.

The result? Back problems can be due to discs that are low in water, and like a tire that has low air, it can eventually blow out or bulge or degenerate. If you aren't hydrating your discs and your joints, you could bend over or twist one day and that joint or disc could blow out.

The popping and creaking of Mary's knees is another example of dehydration. She used to drink a lot of diet sodas, but as she cut back on sodas and increased her water intake (especially alkaline water), the creaking and popping ceased.

Not having enough water is a huge component for those who are battling osteoarthritis. The sodas, coffees, and diet drinks that people drink don't fully count because those drinks are typically caffeinated and have diuretic properties. You need water, a lot of it, to keep your body well hydrated.

Interestingly, I've found that many patients with arthritis, especially rheumatoid arthritis, have pent-up unforgiveness and bitterness locked away inside of them. Letting go of those negative and damaging emotions, including unmet expectations and replacing them with gratitude and hope go a really long way in helping the patients heal.

Fighting pain in your fingers, back, neck, knees, or somewhere else? It is almost always an inflammatory food behind the symptoms, but sometimes it is also related to toxic emotions. Whatever your situation, if you've been wronged, are you willing to let it go?

Years ago, a friend of ours stepped on a piece of wood and got a splinter in her foot. She pulled it out, but her skin didn't properly heal. Finally, after hobbling around for months, she went to a podiatrist. He found an inch-long splinter buried deep in her foot. Once he pulled it out, she quickly healed right up. No more pain.

Remove the "thorn" and your body will heal. That is a message of hope!

THE MODIFIED MEDITERRANEAN DIET FOR ARTHRITIS

How motivated are you to take action? It is really worthwhile to be internally motivated to do whatever it takes to get your health back. If you haven't already, begin by clarifying your "why" for getting healthy. Why do you want to regain your health? Why do you want to beat arthritis?

Work on your answer and refine it until it's a burning white-hot passion that drives you to do whatever it takes to be healthy. Let it propel you to where you want to go, which is a healthy lifestyle that gives you the life and freedom that you want!

Now follows the foundational modified Mediterranean Diet, except in several places you will see that it is altered slightly to best decrease inflammation for arthritis.

Level #1: fruits, vegetables, nuts, beans, and other legumes. Salads consist of dark green leafy lettuce, broccoli, spinach, onions, and cucumbers. Serve vegetables in salads, as appetizers, or as a main or side dish. Fruits are usually a dessert or snack. Use nuts as top-pings to add flavor and texture. The beans and legumes are usu-ally in soups, added to salads, used as dips (i.e., hummus), or as a main dish.

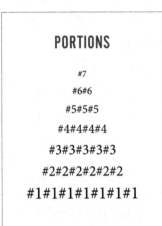

PORTIONS

#7
#6#6
#5#5#5
#4#4#4#4
#3#3#3#3#3
#2#2#2#2#2#2
#1#1#1#1#1#1#1

Altered: Eliminate nightshade plants (tomatoes, eggplant, paprika, pota-toes, and peppers—bell, cayenne, and jalapeno).

Suggestions: Start with a large salad with lunch and dinner (no croutons). Eat vegetables 3 servings a day and more if able. Eat raw, steam, stir-fry, or cook under low heat with olive oil, mac-adamia nut oil, or coconut oil. Eat 1 to 2 servings of fruit a day (blueberries, blackberries, strawberries, raspberries, lemons, limes, or any other types of fruit, but avoid fruit juice).

Suggestions: Eat 1 to 2 cups daily of beans, bean soups, peas, len-tils, legumes, and hummus, preferably before meals. Eliminate soy.

Level #2: steel-cut oats and quinoa, millet or millet bread, brown rice, and sweet potatoes. If you are not gluten sensitive, trying to lose weight, or suffering from high blood pressure, diabetes, or high cholesterol, then potatoes, sprouted bread (i.e., Ezekiel 4:9 bread), or fermented bread (i.e., sourdough bread) are fine on occasion and with moderation, unless you have rheumatoid arthritis.

Altered: Eliminate gluten (wheat, rye, barley) and corn completely from your diet.

Level #3: olive oil, used instead of other oils, margarine, etc. Not only for cooking, it is commonly mixed with balsamic vinegar as a salad dressing.

Altered: Eliminate all fried foods completely from your diet.

Suggestions: Consume 2 to 4 tablespoons of extra-virgin olive oil daily, with cooking and on salads (with balsamic vinegar or any other type of vinegar).

Suggestions: Eat one handful of raw nuts (almonds, hazelnuts, pecans, cashews, walnuts, macadamia) daily.

Level #4: sorry, no dairy.

Altered: Eliminate milk and all dairy completely from your diet.

Altered: Eliminate milk chocolate completely from your diet. Dark chocolate, in moderation, is fine.

Level #5: fish, eaten more than other meats, in about 4- to 6-ounce portions several times a week.

Level #6: chicken, turkey, and eggs without yolks. Chicken in 3- to 6-ounce portions a few times a week is common. The meat is usually skinless and added to soups, stews, and other dishes loaded with vegetables. Only 1 to 6 egg whites per week, 1 egg yolk with 3 egg whites once or twice a week.

Suggestions: If you grill, thinly slice meat and marinate in red wine, juice (pomegranate, cherry), or curry sauce. Remove any char from meat.

Level #7: red meat, in the form of beef, veal, pork, sheep, lamb, and goats, is eaten only a few times a month. It is then often served as a topping to a vegetable, pasta, or rice dish.

Altered: Eliminate beef, pork, and all processed meats completely from your diet.

Suggestions: Rotate vegetables and meats every four days (do not eat the same foods every day). For example, day 1 eat chicken; day 2, turkey; day 3, salmon; and so on.

AUTOIMMUNE DISEASE

An autoimmune disease develops when your immune system attacks healthy cells. One autoimmune disease can attack one or many other types of tissues in the body. Some of the most common autoimmune diseases include:

1. Hashimoto's thyroiditis
2. Rheumatoid arthritis
3. Systemic lupus eurythematosus
4. Graves' disease (overactive thyroid)
5. Type 1 diabetes

6. Inflammatory bowel diseases (Crohn's, ulcerative colitis)

7. Psoriasis

Researchers have identified eighty to one hundred different autoimmune diseases. The National Institue of Health (NIH) estimates that up to 23.5 million Americans have autoimmune diseases, however the NIH numbers only include twenty-four autoimmune diseases. The American Autoimmune Related Disease Association estimates that 50 million Americans suffer from autoimmune diseases.

The cause of autoimmune disease is unknown, however genetics account for approximately half the risk of developing an autoimmune disease and environmental substances account for the remainder. Environmental triggers may be psychological trauma or stress, certain foods, toxins, drugs, heavy metals, pesticides, or nutrient deficiencies such as low vitamin D levels, etc.

I also believe genetically modified foods may be contributing to the rise of autoimmune diseases. A genetically modified organism (GMO) is a plant or animal that has been genetically modified by adding small amounts of genetic material from another organism via molecular techniques. GMO plants have been given genetic traits to protect them from pests, to help them tolerate herbicides (Roundup), or to improve quality. Examples of GMO crops include Roundup Ready soybeans, Roundup Ready corn, Bt potatoes, Bt corn, and more. Some researchers are concerned that the key ingredient in Roundup (glyphosate) interrupts your gut bacteria's metabolic pathways the same way it does a plant, and this may lead to systemic low-grade inflammation. Low-grade systemic inflammation is at the root of most autoimmune diseases.

The American Academy of Environmental Medicine reported, "Several animal studies indicate serious health risks associated with GM food consumption including infertility, immune [problems], accelerated aging, [faulty] insulin regulation, . . . and changes in the liver, kidney, spleen and gastrointestinal system."[14]

Some researchers claim that as many as 70 to 85 percent of the foods sold in grocery stores contain GMOs. However, the FDA does not require companies to divulge on the label whether their foods are GMOs. The seven foods listed below are almost always GMO and, therefore, one should choose organic foods, which do not contain GMOs.

The modified Mediterranean Diet for autoimmune disease is

TOP 7 GMO FOODS[15]

1. Corn (88%)—popular ingredient in processed food and a staple of animal feed
2. Soy (93%)—hydrogenated oils, lecithin, emulsifiers, tocopherol (a vitamin E supplement), and proteins
3. Cottonseed (94%)—vegetable oil, margarine or shortening production, fried foods such as potato chips
4. Canola (90%)—canola oil is used in cooking, as well as biofuels
5. Sugar beets (90%)—sugar beets produce 54% of sugar sold in US
6. Papaya (75% of Hawaiian papaya crop)
7. Alfalfa—no GMO alfalfa on market, but farmers feed it to dairy cows

---

the same as the modified Mediterranean Diet for arthritis, except one should also eliminate all GMO foods, especially GMO corn, soy, cottonseed oil, soybean oil, sugar beets, papaya, and potatoes.

GETTING DOWN TO BUSINESS

The X-rays left no room for doubt. My friend had severe osteoarthritis in his knees. His doctor told him, "You are going to need bilateral total knee replacements. You almost have bone rubbing on bone, which means you have very little cartilage left in your knees at all."

My friend was in his mid-forties and had a lot of life ahead of him yet. The prognosis of two total knee replacements was not the news he had hoped to hear.

When he visited my offices, we analyzed his diet. One thing I noticed right away was his penchant for milk. He loved it and would drink half a gallon of milk every day. As we ran tests, it turned out that he was highly sensitive to dairy.

It also meant that he had been ignoring the warning light of pain that his body had been giving him for quite some time. The persistent pain in his knees was there long before he went to the doctor who did the X-rays and told him his grim news.

The high sensitivity to dairy meant that he was not allergic, but it was certainly causing inflammation, pain, and damage. Right away, he cut out milk, cheese, ice cream, and yogurt completely from his diet. All things dairy were put on hold for twelve months.

At the end of the full year, my friend went back to his orthopedic doctor and said, "Can you look at my knees again?"

His doctor X-rayed both knees, but when they discussed the X-rays, the doctor said, "These can't be the same knees. Last year, you had almost bone on bone, but these knees, the X-rays show, are normal knees. The cartilage has regrown. These simply cannot be the same knees."

My friend laughed. "Oh, it's me. I simply quit eating dairy for twelve months."

Today, many years later, my friend is still the proud owner of two knees that have never been replaced. They are doing fine, and he is doing great as well, but he still avoids dairy.

Thankfully, we were able to get to the bottom of his symptoms and deal with the inflammation.

You can do the same. If your body is blinking that red light of "pain" somewhere, don't ignore it. Find the cause, so that you, like my friend, can truly move on.

CHAPTER EIGHT

℞

YOUR JOURNEY

Chapter Eight is all about type 2 diabetes, knowing what it is and why you certainly don't want it. Instead of following the national trends, you can fight back. Discover precisely how to cure, control, or manage the disease. The process works. It has been proven time and time again. With the modified Mediterranean Diet, you can beat it.

Don Colbert, MD

BEAT TYPE 2 DIABETES
with the Modified Mediterranean Diet

CHUCK WAS A BIT OF an old codger. At age eighty-five, he was set in his ways. His son, in his late fifties, did most of the talking. "The doctor said that Dad is pre-diabetic," he explained. "His hemoglobin A1C level is 6.4."

We both knew that when the hemoglobin A1C levels passed 6.5, he would shift from pre-diabetic to full-on type 2 diabetes. Since the HbA1C level reflects blood sugar levels, the higher the number goes means that the body is becoming more and more resistant to insulin. With type 1 diabetes, the body no longer produces insulin; with type 2 diabetes, the body is producing insulin, but the insulin is not lowering the blood sugar effectively as the body is insulin resistant. Chuck was knocking on the door of a life he did not want to live! Sure, he was old, but this was no way to finish.

"I want to drink what I want and eat what I want," Chuck demanded.

"That means ice cream at nights and donuts for breakfast," his son translated. "I've told him for years that it's not good for him, but he doesn't listen to me."

I whispered to the son, "We need to get your dad to shift his thinking or he is going to eventually destroy his kidneys. Those

HbA1C numbers are already not looking good, and his kidney functions are getting worse."

Chuck was a crusty old man and he needed something that would open his eyes to where he was heading . . . before he got there.

Quite matter-of-factly, I turned to Chuck and stated, "I want you to go to a dialysis unit at a local hospital. The way you are going, you are going to be on dialysis three days a week for three hours a day. For those three hours, you will sit in a chair while they dialyze your blood. Your kidneys will need this because at this rate your kidneys will eventually not function adequately."

I paused and asked, "Are you sure you want to spend three hours a day, three days a week, doing this? I know you have better things to do with your time."

Three short weeks later, the son called and said, "It's like you hit my dad with a two-by-four. He's not eating ice cream at night, he stopped eating donuts for breakfast, and he is already losing belly fat."

FOODS THAT USUALLY RAISE BLOOD SUGAR

- White rice
- Wheat products (bread, pasta, crackers, pretzels, most cereals)
- Processed corn products (corn chips, popcorn, tortillas, corn flour)
- Potatoes, French fries, chips
- Cakes, pies, cookies
- Sodas, sweetened drinks, fruit drinks, smoothies
- Dried fruit

"That is great news," I encouraged.

"But that's not all," the son went on. "He is constantly telling me, 'I am not going to be on dialysis, not a chance!' Thank you for what you told him. It was like a wake-up call."

Being the set-in-his-ways type of guy that Chuck is, I would bet that he will never, ever become type 2 diabetic. I still check his HbA1C numbers every three months and he is doing great.

That is the right type of stubbornness!

MORE THAN A POKE IN THE EYE

The CDC reports that from 1980–2011, the number of people with type 2 diabetes tripled, and that means that today one in eleven people have diabetes and one in three are pre-diabetic. Top it off with a 50 percent increased mortality rate from diabetes and those with type 2 diabetes have a very dark future ahead of them.

According to the American Diabetes Association, complications for those with type 2 diabetes include:

- Skin issues
- Eye issues, including diabetic retinopathy and blindness
- Neuropathy (nerve damage)
- Foot issues, including amputation
- DKA (ketoacidosis)
- Kidney disease (nephropathy)
- High blood pressure
- Stroke
- Hyperosmolar hyperglycemic nonketotic syndrome (HHNS)
- Gastroparesis
- Heart disease

- Mental health issues
- Pregnancy issues

FOODS THAT USUALLY LOWER BLOOD SUGAR

- Steel-cut oatmeal
- Soluble fiber (beans, peas, lentils, hummus)
- Seeds (flax, chia, salba)
- Broccoli, cabbage, brussels sprouts
- Olive oil, avocados
- Almonds, walnuts, cashews
- Dark green leafy vegetables (kale, spinach)

Having type 2 diabetes is not a trivial detail, something you can just ignore or deal with on the weekends or worry about at holidays. The wrinkles, blindness, amputation of limbs, kidney disease, and increased chance for dementia (two to three times more likely) alone are not "minor" details, and they are very real and constant concerns.

This is serious stuff!

With type 2 diabetes, the longer you have it, the greater your risk for these complications striking home. Long-term, unmanaged, high blood-sugar levels mean you are damaging your beta cells that produce insulin. Eventually you will probably need insulin, especially if this has been going on for ten years or longer.

Thankfully, if caught early enough, it's possible to re-sensitize the insulin receptors in your pancreas so that you probably won't need insulin at all, and many can be weaned off their diabetic medicines.

Insulin is like a key that opens the cells to take in the sugar. With insulin resistance, figuratively speaking, the lock is rusty and the key cannot open it. This insulin resistance means you need more and more insulin for sugar to get inside the cell and eventually the body becomes so resistant to insulin that sugar can't get inside the cells and it stays in the blood. You then develop symptoms of increased thirst and increased urination due to elevated sugar in the blood.

If you have had poorly controlled type 2 diabetes for fifteen to twenty years, the damage to the beta cells may be irreversible.

Thankfully, we can still help. You may need to be on a little insulin for the rest of your life due to the damage, but a little insulin is better than a lot.

Remember the stat earlier (from the CDC) about 70 percent of adults being overweight and over 35 percent being obese, and how obesity rates have doubled among adults and children and tripled among adolescents? Quite clearly, the diabetes epidemic is simply following the obesity epidemic.

> **HEALTH**
>
> Your HbA1C number should be 5.6 or less, optimally at 5.0. Do you know your HbA1C number?

Thankfully, this is a statistic that you don't need to live with.

I have seen patients with advanced cancers and people with amyotrophic lateral sclerosis (ALS, or better known as Lou Gehrig's disease). Call me crazy, but when someone comes into my offices with type 2 diabetes, I sometimes laugh. Now, I'm not laughing because I'm rude or insensitive, but because we can beat this thing! If they have had it less than ten years and are not five hundred pounds, we can usually reverse it for most of them.

Thankfully, type 2 diabetes is easy to fix. It's easy to reverse.

HOW YOU CAN FIX YOUR DIABETES

Thankfully, there are answers that can control, manage, and even cure your type 2 diabetes! There is one catch: *you*. That is because you don't *catch* type 2 diabetes . . . you *develop* it over time.

It's yours. You did it. You chose it by consistently making wrong food choices. But you can fix it!

Thankfully, you can get rid of type 2 diabetes that has been rattling like a metal chain around your neck. You can beat it!

I will let the cat out of the bag and give you the three secrets to beating type 2 diabetes. Are you ready? Here they are:

1. Lose belly fat
2. Control your diet
3. Exercise regularly

Armed with that, you will probably never develop type 2 diabetes or can usually reverse it entirely.

> ## HEALTH
>
> Type 3 diabetes, which involves insulin resistance in the brain, is best known by its other name: Alzheimer's disease.

This disease follows your waistline and the answer is the modified Mediterranean Diet. Through it you can lose the belly fat, control your food intake, and nourish your body. All of this will, among many other good things, help re-sensitize your insulin receptors, which will help control your appetite and usually erase the need for insulin shots.

The epidemic of type 2 diabetes is really all about one thing, and one thing alone: *your waistline.*

Right now, measure your waist at the navel. What's your number?

A good number would be half your height, and that holds true if you are a man or a woman. If you are 5 feet 6 inches tall (66 inches), then 33 inches would be the maximum waist size for you. If you are 6 feet tall (72 inches), then 36 inches would be the maximum waist size for you.

These days, the average man's waist size is 38 inches and the average woman's waist size is 35 inches. Here is where things get scary: once a man's waist hits 40 inches and a woman's waist hits 35 inches, they are most often already pre-diabetic!

Because diabetes is a "choice" disease (bad food choices, bad beverage choices, and bad exercise choices), you can also choose to change your mind!

That's right. It was your choice before and it's your choice now. It's always your choice, which means *you* are the one with the power. You can choose, this very moment, to make good food choices.

I have helped many of my patients overcome type 2 diabetes. The modified Mediterranean Diet is the key. Quite sim-

> ### CRAVINGS
>
> Those with type 2 diabetes typically crave:
>
> - sugars
> - processed foods
> - starches
> - wheat
> - corn

ply, patients eliminate sugars, soda, and grains, except for steel-cut oatmeal, and they use beans, peas, and lentils. They decrease their fruit intake, restricting it to blackberries, blueberries, strawberries, raspberries, lemons, and limes.

If they are on medications, I do not suggest that they get off the medications right away, but I do have them track their blood sugar levels daily. However, after a few months, they are usually able to go off one or more of their medications.

Within a few short months, their blood sugar levels usually come down beautifully. If not, they may have to eliminate oats and fruits for a season until their numbers come down. Some nutritional supplements can also be added to speed this up.

With type 2 diabetic patients, if caught soon enough, the cure rate is usually over 90 percent, and it's mainly their diet that they adjust.

Again, it's their choice.

Do you really want to go down the road of type 2 diabetes?

I didn't think so. It's time to get off.

Thankfully, you can.

FOODS THAT USUALLY RAISE TRIGLYCERIDES

- Simple sugars (fructose, sucrose, glucose, corn syrup, honey, maltose, maple syrup, agave nectar)
- Saturated fats (fried foods, red meat, processed meats, chicken skin, high-fat dairy, butter, lard, many fast foods)
- Trans fats (margarine, shortening, many fast foods)
- Refined grains (white bread, wheat bread, pasta, bagels, pretzels, most cereals, instant rice, bagels, pizza)
- Corn products (corn chips, corn tortillas, corn flour, popcorn)
- Starchy foods (potatoes, French fries, potato chips)
- Cakes, pies, cookies, candies, sodas, smoothies, fruit juice

---

THE MODIFIED MEDITERRANEAN DIET FOR DIABETES

How motivated are you to take action? It is really worth it to be internally motivated to do whatever it takes to get your health back.

If you haven't already, begin by clarifying your "why" for getting healthy. Why do you want to regain your health? Why do you want to beat type 2 diabetes?

Work on your answer, refine it until it's a burning white-hot passion that drives you to do whatever it takes to be healthy. Let it propel you to where you want to go, which is a healthy lifestyle that gives you the life and freedom that you want! Do you want to stay healthy and help your children, grandchildren, and great-grandchildren grow up? That's not really even a question, so let's make wise decisions today.

Now follows the foundational modified Mediterranean Diet, except in several places you will see that it is altered slightly to best overcome your type 2 diabetes.

Level #1: fruits, vegetables, nuts, beans, and other legumes. Salads consist of dark green leafy lettuce, fresh vine-ripened tomatoes, broccoli, spinach, peppers, onions, and cucumbers. Serve vegetables in salads, as appetizers, or as a main or side dish. Fruits are usually a dessert or snack. Use nuts as toppings to add flavor and texture. The beans and legumes are usually in soups, added to salads, used as dips (i.e., hummus), or as a main dish.

> *Suggestions:* Start with a large salad with lunch and dinner (no croutons). Eat vegetables 3 servings a day and more if able. Eat raw, steam, stir-fry, or cook under low heat with olive oil, macadamia nut oil, or coconut oil. Eat 1 to 2 servings of fruit a day (blueberries, blackberries, strawberries, raspberries, lemons, and limes—but avoid fruit juice) unless they raise your blood sugar excessively.

Suggestions: Eat 1 to 2 cups daily of beans, bean soups, peas, lentils, legumes, and hummus, preferably before meals. (Before eating beans, you may need to use 2 to 3 Beano tabs to aid with digestion, or soak your beans overnight and discard the water in the morning.)

Level #2: steel-cut oats and quinoa, millet or millet bread, brown rice, and sweet potatoes. If you are not gluten sensitive, trying to lose weight, or suffering from high blood pressure, diabetes, or high cholesterol, then potatoes, sprouted bread (i.e., Ezekiel 4:9 bread), or fermented bread (i.e., sourdough bread) are fine on occasion and with moderation.

Altered: Eliminate gluten (wheat, rye, barley), corn, and white rice completely from your diet. Also eliminate millet, brown rice, and sweet potatoes until the blood sugar is controlled, then limit serving size to the size of a tennis ball.

Level #3: olive oil, used instead of other oils, margarine, etc. Not only for cooking, it is commonly mixed with balsamic vinegar as a salad dressing. Use of small amounts of organic butter is fine.

Altered: Eliminate all fried foods completely from your diet.

Suggestions: Consume 2 to 4 tablespoons of extra-virgin olive oil daily, with cooking and on salads (with balsamic vinegar or any other type of vinegar).

Suggestions: Eat one handful of raw nuts (almonds, hazelnuts, pecans, cashews, walnuts, macadamia) daily.

Level #4: cheese and yogurt, in small amounts. Freshly grated Parmesan on pasta or a little feta cheese on a salad is common. Yogurt (about a cup a day) is how milk is usually eaten, and it is low fat or nonfat, served with fresh fruit added. Yogurt is also a salad dressing (i.e., mixed with cucumbers, garlic, onion, and dill).

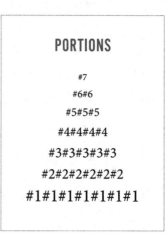

PORTIONS

#7
#6#6
#5#5#5
#4#4#4#4
#3#3#3#3#3
#2#2#2#2#2#2
#1#1#1#1#1#1#1

Altered: May use unsweetened low-fat yogurt or unsweetened low-fat cottage cheese, and add your own fruit (berries), rotating the dairy every 4 days.

Level #5: fish, eaten more than other meats, in about 4- to 6-ounce portions several times a week.

Altered: Eat the lowest mercury fish possible. See Appendix C for list of fish.

Level #6: chicken, turkey, and eggs. Chicken in 3- to 6-ounce portions a few times a week is common. The meat is usually skinless and added to soups, stews, and other dishes loaded with vegetables. Only 1 to 6 eggs per week with 1 egg yolk/3 egg white ratio.

Level #7: red meat, in the form of beef, veal, pork, sheep, lamb, and goats, is eaten only a few times a month. It is then often served as a topping to a vegetable, pasta, or rice dish.

Altered: Eliminate organ meats completely from your diet.

Avoid red meat, pork, lamb, and veal or minimize to 3 to 6 ounces twice a week.

Altered: Eliminate sugar completely from your diet.

Suggestions: Rotate vegetables and meats every 4 days (do not eat the same foods every day). For example, day 1 eat chicken; day 2, turkey; day 3, salmon; and so on.

FOODS THAT USUALLY LOWER TRIGLYCERIDES

- Omega-3 fatty acids (wild salmon, wild sardines)
- Seeds (flax, chia, salba, psyllium)
- Soluble fiber (beans, peas, legumes, lentils, hummus)
- Kale, spinach, leafy greens
- Steel-cut oats
- Broccoli, cabbage
- Berries (blackberries, blueberries, raspberries, strawberries)

TAKING THE NEXT STEPS TO HEALTH

The majority of people in the United States and other Western countries die from diseases of affluence. We have the highest rates of heart diseases, cancers, and diabetes, diseases that typically come as a result of our wealth and food choices.

If you were to catch me on an elevator and ask me for a thirty-second summary on how to beat diabetes, I would say, "You need to lower your blood sugar levels by following the anti-inflammatory modified Mediterranean Diet. Lay off sugar, fruit juice, bread, pasta, crackers, and all wheat and corn products. Walk briskly thirty minutes a day, five to six days a week, lose belly fat to at least half your height in inches, and balance your hormones. Do that and I would bet that your blood sugar will be in the normal range."

Ding! The elevator door opens and you step out.

You have the answers. You've just read it. Are you going to follow through?

If you have type 2 diabetes, you need a wake-up call. As we have discussed, you *catch* a cold and you *catch* the flu, but you *develop* type 2 diabetes by consistently making the wrong food choices. And as I have said many times, genetics load the gun, but bad food choices pull the trigger.

Have you ever seen someone die horribly from type 2 diabetes? If so, that can be a wake-up call.

Have you ever been to a dialysis unit, an amputee ward, a dementia ward, or to the coronary unit where severe congestive heart failure forces patients to be on oxygen for the rest of their lives? If so, that may be a wake-up call.

You need your own "aha" moment when you stubbornly proclaim, "There is no way that is going to happen to me!"

What's it going to take for you? What is the button to push to get you to take action? We all have a trigger. What is yours? What trigger would cause you to take massive action toward a healthy, diabetes-free life?

With that in mind, here is an interesting thought: *You can push your own button.*

You don't need someone else to push your button. You can push it yourself! That is what personal motivation is all about. Find your trigger button and push it!

Hope is right here for you. Nothing we eat is worth dying for.

You may have heard of the term "epigenetics," which focuses on your inherited genes. Certain genes, researchers have found, may be inherited but are activated by your diet, lifestyle, environment, beliefs, and attitude. The turning on or turning off of these certain genes is up to you.

When Jim came to see me, he had decided that enough was enough. He had struggled with type 2 diabetes for almost fifteen years and he couldn't take it anymore. His HbA1C numbers were always over 7.0.

One side effect that he hated the most was that he was perpetually exhausted, always tired, and with no energy. I put him on the modified Mediterranean Diet and helped him clarify which foods would negatively affect his blood sugar levels.

Six months later, his HbA1C number was 5.3, a far cry from the minimal 6.5 for someone with diabetes! He was well within range of "normal," a place he had not been in many years.

He had lost weight and his energy levels were way back up. "I feel great!" he told me.

He left my office a very happy man!

One of the first things he did was schedule a visit with his life insurance company. I guess paying that extra cost as a diabetic was something he wanted to avoid! They also did his blood work, as part of their normal procedure, and contacted him a few days later. They then informed him that he was no longer diabetic.

Jim totally reversed his type 2 diabetes, and it stayed reversed.

You can usually do the same.

CHAPTER NINE

R⃒

YOUR JOURNEY

Chapter Nine is all about the "c-word," cancer. Did you know that cancer is a sugar feeder? With the modified Mediterranean Diet, and some other adjustments, we can create in your body the best environment to starve the very cancer that is hurting you. And when cancer cannot grow, you can often beat it or live with it.

Don Colbert, MD

FIGHTING CANCER
(STAGES 1–2 AND 3–4)
with the Modified Mediterranean Diet

"WE NEED TO REMOVE YOUR KIDNEY," the oncologist explained. "The cancer is aggressive, and the only way to get ahead of it is to remove the kidney, where the cancer is."

Susan was willing, but her husband didn't want to pursue that option just yet. Once that surgery was done, there was no going back.

When they came to see me, they were running out of options and they were running out of time. Because hers was a stage 1 cancer and she refused to have her kidney removed, I put her on a much more radical diet, exercise program, and supplement regimen.

After a few months, she returned to her oncologist. He was amazed at what he found. "I ordered the original biopsy myself, so I know it was an aggressive cancer," he noted, "but the cancer has stopped growing. It's still there, smaller in size, but it's no longer aggressive."

That was great news for both of them!

It has been many years since we first met, and Susan has been living with cancer the entire time. Every three to six months she gets an ultrasound or CT scan done. The cancer has encapsulated itself and is not growing at all. It's basically sitting there, minding its own business, but because of where it is, they don't want to remove it as that would mean removing the kidney as well. By keeping her immune system strong, sticking to the diet, and exercising, she is alive and well.

Eventually, when it is available, Susan will no doubt agree to immunotherapy, which uses her own immune system to attack the tumor.

The non-growing cancer is what I call a "happy cancer," a cancer that we can live with. It is content to just sit there and not grow, having been brought under control.

Now, of course it would have been ideal if the cancer disappeared completely, but it didn't happen. Susan came in with a seriously aggressive cancer, one that did not give her a very big chance of survival, and today she has a bright future ahead of her, even though she still has cancer.

People learn to live with diabetes, arthritis, or heart disease. Now, thanks to the power of diet, you can, if need be, learn to live with cancer as well!

How advanced is advanced?

Cancer ranks as the second highest cause of death in the United States, according to the CDC. In descending order, the most common cancers hitting us at home (says the American Cancer Society Facts and Figures annual report for 2012) include:

1. Skin
2. Lung
3. Prostate
4. Breast

5. Colon
6. Kidney
7. Bladder

That means that one in four deaths in America from cancer is most likely in one of these seven areas . . . at a rate of more than one death per minute!

Prevention is always the goal, as that not only saves lives, it also saves money, time, family loss, job loss, resources, and much more. It would seem obvious that we would try to avoid that which makes us sick, but that is certainly not the case, as the American Cancer Society points out:

- *Preventable*: a third of cancer deaths are caused by tobacco smoking
- *Preventable*: another third of the cancer cases are related to overweight/obesity, physical inactivity, and/or poor nutrition
- *Preventable*: more than three million skin cancer cases per year in the United States are from excessive sun exposure/ indoor tanning

But as we have discussed, prevention requires change at the level of personal choices, and that means we have to decide today how we want to live tomorrow. Sometimes, it is too late.

The Agency for Healthcare Research and Quality puts the direct medical costs for cancer in the United States at around $90 billion per year, and that's not going to be turned around in an instant. It's going to take time.

In fact, it's also going to take a generation of people who are sick of being sick and they fight back by doing what it takes to get healthy, be healthy, and remain healthy. That is another reason the modified Mediterranean Diet is so perfect; it is ideal for today and it is ideal for tomorrow.

As for the cancers, most are discovered at the stage 1 or stage 2 levels, and the good news is that cancer at stage 1 or 2 is treatable. At this level, it is very treatable and curable, and that is very encouraging news—as it should be! I do refer all cancer patients to an oncologist at cutting edge hospitals such as MD Anderson Cancer Center in Houston. I believe that immunotherapy will be the main cancer therapy in the future.

FOODS THAT USUALLY FEED CANCER

- Sugar (cakes, pies, cookies, sodas, candies)
- Polyunsaturated fats (corn oil, safflower oil, soybean oil, cottonseed oil)
- Trans fats (margarine, shortening) and fried foods
- Wheat, corn, white rice
- Alcohol
- Refined processed foods, crackers, bagels, most cereals, chips
- Excessive animal protein (red meat, pork, lamb, veal, and even excessive chicken)

For stage 1 and 2 cancer patients, the best place to begin is with the modified Mediterranean Diet, along with supplements and exercise. I have patients eliminate their problem foods and avoid sugars, avoid or minimize corn and gluten, and avoid breads.

If you have a more advanced cancer (stages 3 or 4), then we need to turn things up a notch. I have developed a special diet that is incredibly effective for patients with stage 3 or stage 4 cancer.

Is all of this guaranteed to cure your cancer? No, nothing is 100 percent guaranteed. But it does help, and we have helped hundreds of patients treat (manage or control) their cancer.

Ideally, you will take action now if you are at the stage 1 or stage 2 level, and get on the best anti-inflammatory diet in the world, the modified Mediterranean Diet. By doing so, you are feeding your body what it needs to deal with the cancer and provide health for your body. Usually, this diet is sufficient to get you healthy and on the road to continued great health.

If you are at stage 3 or stage 4, there is still hope! Many of my patients were told . . . *many years ago* . . . by their oncologists, "You have less than a 5 percent chance of being alive five years from now." When they first received that news, they chose to do whatever it took to get well again.

So, whether you are at stage 1, 2, 3, or 4, it's time to do whatever it takes to get your health back. To get there, you need to put your cancer on a diet.

WHY CANCER NEEDS TO BE ON A DIET

The right type of diet usually slows down the cancer. In fact, the right type of diet can sometimes *stop* cancer growth and may even sometimes *reverse* the growth! That is the nutshell reason you need to put your cancer on a diet.

Every doctor would rather treat a slow-growing tumor than a fast-growing one, and in the near future, I believe we will use diet plus immunotherapy (I call it "diet therapy") to beat cancer completely. The diet puts cancer in a weakened state and then the immunotherapy hopefully destroys the cancer. Chemotherapy has been used for years against fast-growing cancer, but it also may weaken or wipe out your immune system. Immunotherapy works on both rapid- and slow-growing cancers without killing your immune system.

But for now, until this medical breakthrough is fully in practice, we use a powerful diet that usually helps to slow or stop your cancer's growth and then hopefully reverses that growth. After that, you can remove the cancer through surgery or leave it in and manage it under the guidance of your oncologist.

CRAVINGS

Those with cancer typically crave:

- Sugars
- Processed foods
- Starches
- Wheat
- Corn

I had a patient a few years ago with an aggressive, baseball-sized cancerous tumor in his colon. He went immediately on our advanced cancer diet. The cancer stopped growing, and it wasn't long before the cancer had shrunk down to about the size of an egg. A surgeon can remove the tumor at that point—which the patient opted to do—and he was cancer free!

Again, for stage 1 or 2 cancer, the modified Mediterranean Diet is a sufficient starting point, but if you have stage 3 or 4, then you will most likely need to get on our advanced cancer diet. The modified Mediterranean Diet is where you will want to eventually end up, but for now, the advanced cancer diet is needed to bring your cancer in line.

Before I explain the details of this advanced cancer diet, it is important that you understand a bit more about how cancer works. Then you will understand why this is so important.

THE #1 FOOD FOR CANCER: SUGAR

The primary source of food for cancer is sugar. That is because most cancers are glycolytic (feeding off sugar). The cancer thrives on the sugars we have in our bodies, and the typical foods we eat are just that . . . sugar. Consider these items we consume:

- White bread: converts to sugar
- Sweets: sugar
- Processed foods: convert to sugar
- Rice: converts to sugar
- Breads: convert to sugar
- Corn: contains and converts to sugar
- Grains: convert to sugar
- Beans, peas, and lentils: convert to sugar
- Fruits: contain sugar
- Fruit juices: contain sugar
- Juiced carrots or beets: contain a lot of sugar
- Starches: convert to sugar
- Dairy: contains sugar

Even healthy breads, good fruits, beans, yogurt, or juiced carrots all effectively feed the very cancer you are trying to kill.

The modified Mediterranean Diet is not high in sugars anyway, but when stage 1 and stage 2 patients get on the diet, we purposefully lower the sugar intake even more. For stage 3 and stage 4 patients, the advanced cancer diet will completely eliminate sugars so that your cancer usually is not able to thrive since we've taken away its primary food: sugar.

THE #2 FOOD FOR CANCER: ANIMAL PROTEIN

The second biggest source of food for cancer is protein. The cancer feeds on the animal proteins we eat, and we typically consume the very proteins that cancer loves.

Decades ago, T. Colin Campbell conducted studies that showed how a high-protein diet increased cancer with his lab rats, but when he placed them on a low-protein diet, the cancers decreased in size. He repeated the process and found it to still be accurate.

More recent studies, such as one by Valter Longo (director of the Longevity Institute at the University of Southern California), found that people on high animal-protein diets (defined as 20 percent or more of daily calories coming from protein) were four times more likely to die from cancer. Lowering the meat consumption decreased cancer risks considerably, as did exchanging the animal proteins for plant proteins.

In the advanced cancer diet for stage 3 and stage 4 cancer patients, I recommend 5–10 percent protein consumption. The proteins need to come mostly from plants, but we do include some animal protein (5 percent maximum) from turkey, chicken, eggs, and salmon, preferably organic or free-range. We also supplement with pea, rice, non-GMO soy, or hemp protein.

For stage 1 and stage 2 patients, the modified Mediterranean Diet is already low in animal proteins, but we usually lower that even more. The less food for your cancer, the better.

FOODS THAT HELP PREVENT CANCER

- Broccoli, cauliflower, brussels sprouts, spinach, kale, cabbage
- Wild salmon, wild trout, wild sardines
- Green tea
- Flax seeds
- Sea vegetables (kelp, dulse, red and brown seaweed)
- Curry
- Apples, citrus fruits (lemons, limes), pomegranates, berries

---

The bottom-line reason for putting your cancer on a diet is to take away anything and everything that fuels the cancer.

From there, we can build.

THE #3 FOOD FOR CANCER: INFLAMMATORY FATS

Keeping fat intake low has been proven to reduce cancer risk, as studies have shown that cultures with the lowest fat consumption also have the lowest incidence of cancer. Trans fats, fried foods, and excessive polyunsaturated fats trigger inflammation in the body. Inflammation has been linked to the transformation of normal cells into cancer cells. Inhibiting inflammation is very important in slowing the growth of cancer. Certain fats, however, do not fuel inflammation, including omega 3 fats and mono-unsaturated fats.

For stage 3 and 4 cancer patients, the ketogenic diet will provide the anti-inflammatory fats to help quench inflammation and defuel your cancer.

THE MODIFIED MEDITERRANEAN DIET
FOR STAGE 1 AND STAGE 2 CANCER

How motivated are you to take action? It is really worthwhile to be internally motivated to do whatever it takes to get your health back. If you haven't already, begin by clarifying your "why" for getting healthy. Why do you want to regain your health? Why do you want to beat your cancer?

Work on your answer and refine it until it's a burning white-hot passion that drives you to do whatever it takes to be healthy. Let it propel you to where you want to go, which is a healthy lifestyle that gives you the life and freedom that you want!

Now follows the foundational modified Mediterranean Diet,

except in several places you will see that it is altered slightly to best decrease your stage 1 or stage 2 cancer.

Level #1: fruits, vegetables, nuts, beans, and other legumes. Salads consist of dark green leafy lettuce, fresh vine-ripened tomatoes, broccoli, spinach, peppers, onions, and cucumbers. Serve vegetables in salads, as appetizers, or as a main or side dish. Fruits are usually a dessert or snack. Use nuts as toppings to add flavor and texture. The beans and legumes are usually in soups, added to salads, used as dips (i.e., hummus), or as a main dish.

PORTIONS

```
            #7
          #6#6
        #5#5#5
      #4#4#4#4
    #3#3#3#3#3
  #2#2#2#2#2#2
#1#1#1#1#1#1#1
```

Suggestions: Start with a large salad with lunch and dinner (no croutons). Eat vegetables 3 servings a day and more if able. Eat raw, steam, stir-fry, or cook under low heat with olive oil, macadamia nut oil, or coconut oil. Eat fruits, 2 or more servings a day (blueberries, blackberries, strawberries, raspberries, lemons, limes, or any other types of fruit, but avoid fruit juice).

Suggestions: Eat 1 to 2 cups daily of beans, bean soups, peas, lentils, legumes, and hummus, preferably before meals. Eliminate all GMO soy.

Level #2: steel-cut oats and quinoa, millet or millet bread, brown rice, brown rice pasta, and sweet potatoes. If you are not gluten sensitive, trying to lose weight, or suffering from high blood pressure, diabetes, or high cholesterol, then potatoes, sprouted bread (i.e.,

Ezekiel 4:9 bread), or fermented bread (i.e., sourdough bread) are fine on occasion and with moderation.

Altered: Limit or eliminate gluten (wheat, barley, and rye), corn, and white rice from your diet. If you do eat these, eat small servings for breakfast or lunch and rotate the food no more often than every four days. Limit servings to the size of a tennis ball.

Level #3: olive oil, used instead of other oils, margarine, etc. Not only for cooking, it is commonly mixed with balsamic vinegar as a salad dressing. Small amounts of organic butter are fine.

Altered: Eliminate all fried foods completely from your diet.

Suggestions: Consume 2 to 4 tablespoons of extra-virgin olive oil daily, with cooking and on salads (with balsamic vinegar or any other type of vinegar).

Suggestions: Eat one handful of raw nuts (almonds, hazelnuts, pecans, cashews, walnuts, macadamia) daily.

Level #4: cheese and yogurt, in small amounts. Freshly grated Parmesan on pasta or a little feta cheese on a salad is common. Yogurt (about a cup a day) is how milk is usually eaten, and it is low fat or nonfat, served with fresh fruit added. Yogurt is also a salad dressing (i.e., mixed with dill, garlic, onion, and cucumbers).

Altered: May use low-fat yogurt or unsweetened low-fat cottage cheese, and add your own fruit, rotating the dairy every four days.

Level #5: fish, eaten more than other meats, in about 4- to 6-ounce portions several times a week.

> *Altered:* Eat the lowest mercury fish possible. (See Appendix C for list of fish.)

Level #6: organic or free-range chicken, turkey, and eggs. Chicken in 3- to 4-ounce portions a few times a week is common. The meat is usually skinless and added to soups, stews, and other dishes loaded with vegetables. Only 1 to 6 eggs per week with 1 egg yolk/3 egg white ratio.

> *Suggestions:* If you grill, thinly slice meat and marinate in red wine, juice (pomegranate, cherry), or curry sauce. Remove any char from meat.

Level #7: red meat, in the form of beef, veal, pork, sheep, lamb, and goats, is eaten only a few times a month. It is then often served as a topping to a vegetable, pasta, or rice dish.

> *Altered:* Eliminate pork, lamb, veal, and organ meats completely from your diet. Avoid red meat or minimize to 3 to 4 ounces once or twice a week.

> *Altered:* Eliminate sugar completely from your diet.

> *Suggestions:* Rotate vegetables and meats every four days (do not eat the same foods every day). For example, day 1, eat chicken; day 2, turkey; day 3, salmon; and so on.

THE ADVANCED CANCER DIET
FOR STAGE 3 AND STAGE 4 CANCER

The diet for stage 3 or stage 4 cancer is a more strict diet than the modified Mediterranean Diet.

Just as motivation is required for the modified Mediterranean Diet, which is ideal for stage 1 and stage 2 cancer patients, so even more motivation is required for the advanced cancer diet. In fact, this diet requires greater effort and greater sacrifice.

Are you willing to sacrifice all sugars, starches, and grains to live?

Are you willing to shift your diet radically?

Are you willing to do whatever it takes to get your health back?

Those are important questions to answer. If patients tell me they are not willing to deny themselves in order to live, then I have to tell them, "Thank you for being honest, but I really can't help you if you won't help yourself."

But if you are willing, then so am I! And when you put your mind to it, you will be amazed at how a strong mental attitude will prove to be beneficial!

Are you willing to change your diet so we can boost your immune system?

Are you willing to eliminate certain foods in order to begin starving your cancer?

Are you willing to spice this diet up and make it as palatable as possible?

Great! Then let's do it, together. You may not realize this, but there is an army of supporters around you. Many will link arms with you—just ask them! You will be surprised how many people will support you, believe in you, pray for you, and encourage you.

You may have been wondering, "If we are shifting the body *away* from the sugars that the cancer is eating, what are we shifting the body *to*? What exactly *is* my body going to live on and what *am* I going to eat?"

The answers are exactly what make this diet so powerful for cancer patients.

The advanced cancer diet is ketogenic in nature. That means your body shifts from burning sugars to burning ketone bodies, which are fats. Since most cancers thrive on sugars but cannot thrive on ketone bodies, you are basically smothering the flames of cancer. Throwing sand on the fire, dousing it with water, spraying it with your fire extinguisher—you name it, that's what you are doing!

Without sugar, the cancer's primary fuel supply, the cancer usually cannot effectively grow. Through the advanced cancer diet, we get your body into mild to moderate ketosis, and your body usually thrives eventually, but the cancer does not get its preferred choice of fuel and instead of thriving, often it simply tries to survive.

You have started to turn the tables on your cancer!

A sixty-seven-year-old woman came in with stage 4 ovarian cancer. "I'll do anything to live," she said. "My doctors have given me less than a 10 percent chance to make it five years."

She got on the ketogenic diet, which literally took the fuel away from her cancer, and the cancer shrank significantly. She learned to live with the cancer, and her five-year mark has long since come and gone.

Remember how the number one food for cancer is sugar and the number two food is protein? Those come into play here, for we eliminate sugar and feed your body the right type of proteins and plenty of anti-inflammatory vegetables when you are on the ketogenic diet.

In addition to eliminating sugars and feeding your body the right proteins, the ketogenic diet is one more thing: it is high in healthy fats.

That is what your body will burn: ketones, which are fats. The cancer usually cannot thrive on fats, but you can.

Dr. Thomas Seyfried has done *a lot* of research on the ketogenic diet in mice and has found that it slows down stage 3 and stage 4 advanced cancers.[16] The diet for humans should consist of 80 percent fats, with small amounts of protein, and low-carb, non-starchy vegetables. He found that he could shift the metabolism from burning sugars to burning fats, and since cancers are not metabolically engineered to burn fats, the diet effectively slowed aggressive growth, new blood vessels, and tumor growth.

Interestingly, Dr. Seyfried used polyunsaturated fats, which at excessive amounts are inflammatory. Still, by taking away the main fuel supply (sugar), the cancer couldn't thrive. But I've found that by using healthy fats the results are usually even better.

I have tweaked and revised the ketogenic diet for my patients to be based on these percentages and include these foods:

- *80 percent healthy fats*: coconut oil, MCT coconut oil, flaxseed oil, extra-virgin olive oil, avocados, almond butter, avocado oil, raw nuts such as almonds, pecans, walnuts, and macadamia nuts, and seeds such as flax seeds, chia seeds, salba seeds, hemp seeds, and psyllium seeds (nut butter and seeds ground up in a coffee grinder are more easily digested than eating whole nuts and seeds)
- *15 percent greens*: green vegetables such as spinach, kale, romaine, broccoli, asparagus, cabbage, artichoke, arugula, bok choy, brussels sprouts, cauliflower, celery, chard, chives,

onions, collard greens, garlic, green beans, lettuce, mustard greens, olives, scallions, string beans, watercress, zucchini, sea vegetables (agar, arame, dulse, kombu, nori, sea palm, and wakame), and herbs and spices (basil, black pepper, cardamom, cilantro, garlic, ginger, rosemary, sage, tarragon, thyme, turmeric, and curry)

- *5 percent protein*: most from plant, some animal protein (organic or free-range turkey, chicken, eggs, wild salmon, sardines, trout), and supplement pea, rice, hemp, or non-GMO soy protein

Still no sugar, but combined with healthy fats, healthy proteins, and plenty of greens and supplements, the ketogenic diet is incredibly powerful for stage 3 and stage 4 cancer patients.

UNDERSTANDING YOUR KETOGENIC DIET

Balance is the key to your ketogenic diet. With the right balance, we can maximize the diet's effectiveness against your cancer.

We aim for 80 percent fats, 5 percent protein (up to 10 percent protein, if 5 percent is max protein from animals), and 15 percent plant from non-starchy vegetables. This translates into:

- On a 2,000-calorie-a-day diet, 1,600 calories should come from your good fats and 400 calories from your non-starchy vegetables and protein.
- On a 2,500-calorie-a-day diet, 2,000 calories should come from your good fats and 500 calories from your non-starchy vegetables and proteins.

Great non-starchy vegetables are broccoli, kale, romaine lettuce, spinach, cauliflower, cabbage, asparagus, bean sprouts, avocado, onion, garlic, and bok choy (see list on previous page).

Healthy sources of animal protein are 2 to 3 ounces of organic or free-range chicken, turkey, eggs, or wild salmon, trout, and sardines. Steaming or stir-frying these at low heat with coconut oil is recommended, along with the vegetables above.

Excellent snacks are such things as guacamole with celery sticks, almonds, and almond butter. I also recommend protein drinks two to four times a day, between meals. Those drinks would include:

- ½ to 1 scoop of plant protein
- 1 tablespoon of almond butter
- 1 tablespoon of coconut oil
- 1 tablespoon of flaxseed oil
- 1 tablespoon of extra-virgin olive oil
- 2 tablespoons of ground flax seeds, chia seeds, or salba seeds
- Mix with low sugar almond milk, coconut milk, or water if needed to achieve ketosis (use two or more of the oils in each protein drink)

People with cancer are typically older and digesting nuts can be more difficult, so nut butters are better. These include almond butter, macadamia nut butter, pecan butter, and cashew butters. These monounsaturated fats are healthy fats and usually do not raise your cholesterol levels.

Remember: all sugars are eliminated, which means certain vegetables, such as tomatoes, carrots, and beets, are out because they contain more sugar, and that empowers the cancer. Also avoid eating corn, potatoes, sweet potatoes, most fruit, and rice. Do eat lots of salad with vinegar, extra-virgin olive oil, and garlic. A slice of lemon or lime is fine as long as you remain in ketosis. Healthy ketogenic soups and salads are key to this program.

A comprehensive multivitamin is necessary to make sure that you are getting your daily values of vitamins and minerals. Also a digestive enzyme with adequate lipase is needed by most to help digest the fats. The enzyme should be taken with meals and snacks.

Exercise is also an important part of your balanced diet. Spending fifteen to thirty minutes a day walking briskly is a great place for most patients to start. The goal is to get your heart rate up, strengthen your heart, maintain your muscles, and improve your immune system. Losing unnecessary fat is fine, but not muscle mass.

Another important part of the ketogenic diet includes staying in positive nitrogen balance. This is typically difficult for cancer patients. Healthy and adequate proteins (from plant and animal) and specific amino acids (in the form of supplements) help you stay in positive nitrogen balance. That is critically important.

If you have seen advanced cancer patients who look emaciated or wasted away, that is the result of muscle loss and negative nitrogen balance. The cancer is burning their muscles as fuel to feed itself, and then the muscles atrophy and their immune system falters. But when you are on the ketogenic diet, this usually does not happen because you stop feeding the cancer and start nourishing the body.

Another element of balance involves your pancreatic enzymes. I have found there to be a pancreatic enzyme insufficiency with most of my cancer patients. A good digestive enzyme will help you digest protein and fat. Most patients cannot properly digest the fats, so enzyme supplements with adequate lipase are needed so they don't get diarrhea and lose weight on this high-fat ketogenic diet. Plus, you need to be eating the correct fuel mixture every three to four hours.

A lot of people with cancer have blood clots, and doctors usually prescribe Coumadin as a blood thinner. However, doctors advise patients to avoid green vegetables if they take Coumadin because greens are typically high in vitamin K, which reverses the blood thinning effect of Coumadin. But those green vegetables are an important part of the ketogenic diet, not to mention the normal health benefits of eating vegetables, and that places cancer patients in a double bind. The answer is simple: I put them on a different medication such as Eliquis that prevents blood clots but still allows them to eat and absorb the green vegetables. This is critical.

Once people get in the groove and their bodies reach a steady state of mild to moderate ketosis, they usually feel really good. But it is a one- to four-week process for most people to get there, and they typically feel really tired, forgetful, light-headed, or blah during the transition time. For these reasons I do not recommend that you work a full-time job. You are fighting for your life, and you need your energy for the battle. I am still amazed at how many patients continue to work such long and grueling hours while in the midst of a battle with stage 3 or 4 cancer. This is where having friends, family, caregivers, a life coach, nutrition coach, or support group is so helpful. The encouragement can literally be a lifesaver.

While you are on the ketogenic diet, you need to monitor your weight daily and increase the fat intake or eat more frequently every two to three hours so you don't lose excessive weight. I also recommend that you monitor your ketones daily with inexpensive ketone strips. These measure the ketones in your urine. You can also measure your blood sugar or your blood ketones. Sometimes we have to get blood sugar levels down to 55–65 mg/dl, and when you are that low you may feel terrible at first, but that is why you need to eat every two to four hours. This keeps the blood sugars stable as you stay in mild to moderate ketosis. Dr. Seyfried recommends that you measure both blood and urine ketones. Also, all medication should be closely monitored by your medical doctor since the ketogenic diet can significantly affect dosages.

I prefer that you have your ketogenic diet for cancer supervised by a knowledgeable nutritionist, dietician, or doctor. You also need a good multivitamin and vitamin C, as the diet eliminates most fruits (except lemon or lime) as they contain sugars. Later on, when you reach a steady state of ketosis, a small amount of berries (a handful) can usually be added, provided you stay in ketosis.

When your body shifts to a steady state of ketosis and you are no longer feeding your cancer the sugars it needs, it is as if a cannon has gone off inside of your body! There is a "boom" as the cancer usually begins to shift to survival mode instead of thriving and spreading.

You know what else happens? Your cancer has now most likely become a treatable chronic disease. That is amazing! Now, I cannot say as a doctor that I have cured people of cancer, but I *can* say that the ketogenic diet has enabled many to treat their cancer like it is a chronic disease, such as high blood pressure or diabetes or high cholesterol. They can live with diabetes . . . and now you can live with cancer!

YOU HAVE WHAT IT TAKES!

You are motivated, you are willing, and you have what it takes! I am confident of that.

Making the shift from burning sugars to burning ketones is a major shift, but you can do it. Your motivating reasons for health and life are vitally important at this stage of the game. Yes, it takes time and effort to coordinate and cook, but life is worth it!

Now, if a doctor tells you or a friend, "There is maybe a five percent chance that you will be here in five years," those words no longer hold such fear and dread!

When Sylvia came to see me, she had a look of hopelessness in her eyes; I could see it across her face. She had advanced stage 4 breast cancer that had spread to her bones and lungs. To top it off, her doctor had given her a very short life expectancy of only six months.

As we talked, I caught a few glimmers of hope, little things she would say that she wanted still to do, be, and accomplish in life. I also noticed that it was her husband who quickly stepped in to keep her in line. He was so full of negative "what ifs" that she could hardly breathe. He was practically sucking the hope right out of her.

I told them both to stop magnifying the problem. I also addressed the husband's grasshopper mentality. "Though you are well-intentioned, you are sabotaging your wife's health," I told him. "Let her hope arise, give it a chance, and encourage her."

We talked about the modified Mediterranean Diet and the advanced cancer diet, about inflammation and cancer, and about foods and cooking. I told them how the ketogenic diet had worked with hundreds of other advanced cancer patients.

When they left, she was beaming with joy. She was so full of hope! And that is a beautiful and necessary place to begin.

CHAPTER TEN

℞

YOUR JOURNEY

Chapter Ten is all about the seemingly mystifying dementia diseases, especially Alzheimer's. There is no instant, one-size-fits-all cure, but there is a lot we can do to prevent and treat it, and with amazing results. If you have mild to moderate dementia, in any form, then this chapter is for you. I know you will be encouraged!

Don Colbert, MD

BEAT DEMENTIA AND ALZHEIMER'S

with the Modified Mediterranean Diet

A HUSBAND AND WIFE PASTOR TEAM came to see me several years ago. They were in their early sixties, still very busy and active in the church they had started, but everything had come to a screeching halt. One Sunday, a few months earlier, the wife was preaching and halfway through her sermon she forgot everything she was saying, where she was, and what she was doing.

Naturally, that scared everyone in the congregation. She had to stop preaching, though she enjoyed it and wanted desperately to be back in her role as co-pastor. When her doctor diagnosed her with mild-to-moderate dementia, that seemed to be the end of it.

I asked them my usual 1001 questions, analyzed her diet, and more. It didn't take long to discover that she was eating gluten at every meal. She was also not sleeping at night, was not exercising, was overweight, was not taking any coconut oil, and—among other things—she was on drugs to lower her cholesterol.

We paused as I explained how the brain needs cholesterol. I have had hundreds of patients who have been diagnosed with dementia due to the very drugs they were taking to lower their cholesterol. So many cholesterol drugs interfere with cholesterol synthesis, the key fat for the brain.

We began to make changes. The first thing she did was to get off her cholesterol medication. Her doctor complained, but I told him, "This may be one of the factors that are causing her dementia."

In its place, I put her on a natural supplement to lower bad cholesterol but boost the good cholesterol. I also put her on co-enzyme Q10 and on coconut oil (a teaspoon at meals and at bedtime); checked her B12 levels and her homocysteine level; started her on B12 supplements; lowered her homocysteine level to less than 7; took her off gluten; and put her on the modified Mediterranean Diet. She started exercising fifteen to thirty minutes a day, five days a week. She also cut out MSG and NutraSweet (she was a heavy diet soda drinker). Finally, she made sure her dinner and breakfast were at least twelve hours apart. Yes, fasting helps with memory loss.

CRAVINGS

Those with dementia typically crave:

- Fried foods
- Processed foods (with MSG)
- Drinks (with NutraSweet)
- Breads

Within six months, she was back, in more ways than one. When I first saw her, she had no spark. Her mind and eyes were dull and cloudy. She couldn't focus and her mind wasn't taking in what I was saying. It was as if the lights were not on in her eyes. When she came back through that door six months later, it was like I was meeting a different person! There was a spark in her eyes, she was vivacious, and she was engaging. She talked a mile a minute, happy and full of life.

Her husband was all smiles. He gave me a big hug and said with a voice full of emotion and tears in his eyes, "Thank you. I've got my wife back. Her mind doesn't skip. She's preaching again and she doesn't forget things mid-sentence. We simply did everything you told us to do."

"And my primary care doctor," she added, "cannot believe the results."

Thankfully, early dementia can usually be improved or even reversed with the correct diet, nutritional program, and lifestyle program.

MANY DEMENTIAS, MANY CHALLENGES

Medically speaking, there are more than one hundred different types of dementia, with Alzheimer's by far the most common. The Alzheimer's Association reports that one in three senior citizens will die from Alzheimer's or another form of dementia and that Alzheimer's is now the sixth leading cause of death in the United States.[17] Interestingly, most (almost two-thirds) of the victims are women.

The current global costs for dementia, according to the World Health Organization, top the scales at over US $600 billion per year, and that figure is only going to go up as the number of patients with dementia increases each year.

They say there is no known cure and no way to prevent dementia, but the Mayo Clinic says that it "may be beneficial" to engage in the following:[18]

- *Keep your mind active*: Mentally stimulating activities, such as puzzles and word games, and memory training may delay the onset of dementia and help decrease its effects.
- *Be physically and socially active*: Physical activity and social

interaction may delay the onset of dementia and reduce its symptoms.

- *Quit smoking*: Some studies have shown smoking in middle age and older may increase your risk of dementia and blood vessel (vascular) conditions. Quitting smoking may reduce your risk.
- *Lower your blood pressure*: High blood pressure may lead to a higher risk of some types of dementia. More research is needed to determine whether treating high blood pressure may reduce the risk of dementia.
- *Pursue education*: People who have spent more time in formal education appear to have a lower incidence of mental decline, even when they have brain abnormalities. Researchers believe that education may help your brain develop a strong nerve cell network that compensates for nerve cell damage caused by Alzheimer's disease.
- *Maintain a healthy diet*: Eating a healthy diet is important for many reasons, but a diet rich in fruits, vegetables, and omega-3 fatty acids, commonly found in certain fish and nuts, may promote overall health and lower your risk of developing dementia.

If that's all we had to go on, which most people do, that is a pretty grim prognosis!

FINDING ANSWERS FOR DEMENTIA PATIENTS

Alzheimer's disease was first described about a hundred years ago, but we have yet to come up with an effective treatment for it. For dementia as a whole, I don't think we have found answers for two main reasons:

1. *We are eating the wrong foods*: Our diet is only getting worse, the foods we consume are less and less healthy and more and more inflammatory, and changing our diet is something that few people are willing to do.

2. *The puzzle is complicated*: There are many factors that are interconnected, which means there is no single fix, no single pill that will cure everything all at once.

These two reasons come directly into play when you are dealing with any dementia, not just Alzheimer's.

One study by Dr. Dale Bredesen and the Mary S. Easton Center for Alzheimer's Research[19] found what he believed to be a thirty-six–point therapeutic program for Alzheimer's treatment and prevention. He created a specific regimen that he put his patients through, and he was able to reverse early Alzheimer's in most of his patients.

Some of the factors included sleeping seven to eight hours a night, meditating twice a day to reduce stress, exercising thirty minutes a day four to six times a week, improving oral hygiene (with an electric flosser and an electric toothbrush), and reinstating hormone replacement therapy. Regarding food, he recommended fasting at least twelve hours at night (no food between dinner and breakfast, over a period

---

FOODS THAT USUALLY CONTRIBUTE TO MEMORY LOSS

- Wheat products
- Corn products
- Sugar (cakes, pies, sodas)
- Trans fats/fried foods
- Processed meat, sausages
- Polyunsaturated fats (corn oil, sunflower oil, safflower oil, cottonseed oil)
- Alcohol (beer, spirits, wine)

of twelve hours or more), taking melatonin, methylcobalamin, vitamin D3, fish oil, and coenzyme Q10 each day. Also, taking coconut oil and vitamin B12, eliminating all simple carbohydrates, gluten, and processed foods, and eating vegetables, fruits, and non-farmed fish.

Doing these things brought dramatic changes. Most of his patients were able to go back to their jobs without difficulty, and that is the real proof. I love that, for those are the real needs of patients.

It was confirming to see that much of the food-related elements for dementia patients are addressed with the modified Mediterranean Diet, from which I've been getting similar results for years.

THE MODIFIED MEDITERRANEAN DIET FOR DEMENTIA

How motivated are you to take action? It is really worth it to be internally motivated to do whatever it takes to get your health back. If you haven't already, begin by clarifying your "why" for getting healthy. Why do you want to regain your health? Why do you want to beat dementia and Alzheimer's?

Work on your answer amd refine it until it's a burning white-hot passion that drives you to do whatever it takes to be healthy. Let it propel you to where you want to go, which is a healthy lifestyle that gives you the life and freedom that you want! Do you want to stay healthy and help your children and grandchildren grow up? Do you really want to live out the remainder of your life in a nursing home? That's not really even a question, so let's make wise decisions today.

Now follows the foundational modified Mediterranean Diet, except in several places you will see that it is altered slightly to best overcome dementia or Alzheimer's.

Level #1: fruits, vegetables, nuts, beans, and other legumes. Salads consist of dark green leafy lettuce, fresh vine-ripened tomatoes, broccoli, spinach, peppers, onions, and cucumbers. Serve vegetables in salads, as appetizers, or as a main or side dish. Fruits are usually a dessert or snack. Use nuts as toppings to add flavor and texture. The beans and legumes are usually in soups, added to salads, used as dips (i.e., hummus), or as a main dish.

Suggestions: Start with a large salad with lunch and dinner (no croutons). Eat vegetables 3 servings a day and more if able. Eat raw, steam, stir-fry, or cook under low heat with olive oil, macadamia nut oil, or coconut oil. Eat 2 servings of fruit a day (blueberries, blackberries, strawberries, raspberries, lemons, limes, or any other types of fruit, but avoid fruit juice).

> ## KEY FOODS THAT MAY PREVENT MEMORY LOSS
>
> - Dark chocolate
> - Coconut oil, coconuts
> - Almonds, walnuts, cashews
> - Fresh berries (blueberries, blackberries, strawberries, raspberries)
> - Pomegranates
> - Curry
> - Olive oil
> - avocados

Suggestions: Eat ½ to 2 cups daily of beans, bean soups, peas, lentils, legumes, and hummus, preferably before meals.

Altered: Avoid all GMO soy.

Level #2: steel-cut oats and quinoa, millet or millet bread, brown rice, and sweet potatoes. If you are not gluten sensitive, trying to lose weight, or suffering from high blood pressure, diabetes, or high cholesterol, then potatoes, sprouted bread (i.e., Ezekiel 4:9 bread), or fermented bread (i.e., sourdough bread) are fine on occasion and with moderation.

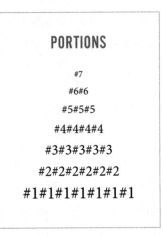

PORTIONS

#7
#6#6
#5#5#5
#4#4#4#4
#3#3#3#3#3
#2#2#2#2#2#2
#1#1#1#1#1#1#1

Altered: Eliminate gluten (wheat, barley, rye), corn, and white rice completely from your diet. Eliminate all processed foods. Limit millet, millet bread, brown rice, and sweet potatoes to the size of a tennis ball, and limit starches to 1 with each meal.

Level #3: olive oil, used instead of other oils, margarine, etc. Not only for cooking, it is commonly mixed with balsamic vinegar as a salad dressing. Small amounts of organic butter are fine.

Altered: Eliminate all fried foods completely from your diet and minimize or avoid polyunsaturated fats (corn oil, cotton seed oil, sunflower oil, safflower oil, soybean oil). Also avoid GMO oils such as most canola oils, and avoid all trans fats and hydrogenated fats.

Suggestions: Consume 2 to 4 tablespoons of extra-virgin olive oil daily, with cooking and on salads (with balsamic vinegar or any other type of vinegar).

Suggestions: Eat one handful of raw nuts (almonds, hazelnuts, pecans, cashews, walnuts, macadamia) daily.

Level #4: cheese and yogurt, in small amounts. Freshly grated Parmesan on pasta or a little feta cheese on a salad is common. Yogurt (about a cup a day) is how milk is usually eaten, and it is low fat or nonfat, served with fresh fruit added. Yogurt is also a salad dressing (i.e., mixed with dill, garlic, onion, and cucumbers).

> *Altered:* May use low-fat yogurt or unsweetened low-fat cottage cheese, and add your own fruit, rotating the dairy every four days.

Level #5: fish, eaten more than other meats, in about 4- to 6-ounce portions several times a week.

> *Altered:* Eat the lowest mercury fish possible. (See Appendix C for list of fish.)

Level #6: organic or free-range chicken, turkey, and eggs. Chicken in 3- to 6-ounce portions a few times a week is common. The meat is usually skinless and added to soups, stews, and other dishes loaded with vegetables. Only 1 to 6 eggs per week with 1 egg yolk/ 3 egg white ratio.

Level #7: organic or free-range red meat, in the form of beef, veal, pork, sheep, lamb, and goats, is eaten only a few times a month. It is then often served as a topping to a vegetable, pasta, or rice dish.

> *Altered:* Eliminate organ meats completely from your diet. Avoid red meat or minimize to 3 to 6 ounces once or twice a week.

Suggestions: Rotate vegetables and meats every four days (do not eat the same foods every day). For example, day 1, eat chicken; day 2, turkey; day 3, salmon; and so on.

GETTING A HANDLE ON *MODERATE* DEMENTIA

If your dementia, or the dementia of a loved one, is past mild and into moderate, then my suggestion is that you move toward a more ketogenic diet. A stage 3–4 cancer patient needs the *strict* ketogenic diet for cancer, but not so with you. A *milder* form of the ketogenic diet is recommended.

Here are the rules of your *mild* ketogenic diet:

- Limit total carb intake to 50–75 grams a day or less.
- Monitor urine ketones in the morning, afternoon, and evening, adjusting carb intake accordingly. Your goal is to have your urine ketones in the small to trace range (slightly pink).
- Avoid all corn, wheat, and sugar products as well as rice, millet, regular oatmeal, and all processed foods.
- Eat a large breakfast, medium lunch, and small dinner.
- Purchase a carb gram counter to add up your daily carb intake.
- Drink plenty of water, sparkling water, tea, or green tea sweetened with stevia; add a slice of lemon or lime if desired.
- Snacks include a handful or more of nuts (pecans, walnuts, cashews, and almonds, best if raw), slices of coconut (handful or more), and small amounts of dark chocolate (low sugar) or dark chocolate-covered coconut slices, avocado, or guacamole.

- Follow sample menu (that follows) and adapt it to your needs.
- Eat 3–6 oz. of sliced chicken or other meat.
- Eat plenty of green vegetables.
- Fast at least twelve hours after eating dinner.

A mild ketogenic diet would look something like this:

BREAKFAST #1:
- Steel-cut oatmeal (1 cup cooked; 21 grams of carbs)
- ¼ cup blackberries, raspberries, strawberries, or blueberries
- Handful of pecans, walnuts, or almonds
- Sweeten with stevia
- 2–3 oz. of wild salmon or 2–3 oz. cottage cheese
- Coffee sweetened with stevia (using low-sugar coconut milk as creamer), green tea sweetened with stevia, or water
- 1 heaping tsp. extra-virgin coconut oil

BREAKFAST #2:
- 3 egg omelet (1 egg yolk, 3 egg whites)
- Add onions, peppers, mushrooms, tomatoes, spinach, avocado, and other vegetables if desired
- May add a small amount of cheese (1 oz. or less) every four days
- ¼ cup blackberries, raspberries, strawberries, blueberries, or Granny Smith apple
- Coffee sweetened with stevia (using coconut milk as creamer), green tea sweetened with stevia, or water
- 1 heaping tsp. extra-virgin coconut oil

LUNCH:

- A large salad with lots of vegetables, and use extra-virgin olive oil and vinegar for dressing, no croutons
- Non-cream-based, low-sodium vegetable soup (without pasta or rice) or black bean soup (½ cup black beans, 13 grams) or lentil soup (½ cup lentils, 12 grams)
- As many steamed, raw, or stir-fried green vegetables as desired
- 3–6 oz. protein (chicken, turkey, fish, with red meat only once or twice a week), and no processed meats
- Water, sparkling water, green tea (with lemon or lime, and stevia to sweeten)
- 1 heaping tsp. extra-virgin coconut oil

DINNER:

- A large salad, with extra-virgin olive oil and vinegar for dressing, no croutons
- Non-cream based, low sodium vegetable soup (without pasta or rice)
- As many steamed, raw, or stir-fried green vegetables as desired
- 3–6 oz. protein (chicken, turkey, fish, with red meat only once or twice a week), and no processed meats
- Water, sparkling water, green tea (with lemon or lime, and stevia to sweeten)
- 1 heaping teaspoon extra-virgin coconut oil

BEDTIME SNACK:

(best to avoid and fast for twelve hours after dinner)

- A few slices of coconut
- 1 tsp. extra-virgin coconut oil

SMOOTHIE RECIPE:

(smoothie can be eaten between meals)

8–12 oz. unsweetened coconut milk or almond milk

1 tsp.–1 tbsp. coconut oil

1 tsp.–1 tbsp. almond butter

½–1 scoop plant protein

Ice if desired

¼ cup frozen blueberries

May add 1–2 tbsp. of ground flaxseeds

It may take one to four weeks before you reach mild ketosis. If you are not in a mild state of ketosis after four weeks, then you should decrease or stop all bean consumption and decrease intake of steel-cut oatmeal to ½ a cup in the morning and limit fruit to just ¼ cup of berries per day. Rarely, some patients need to decrease their carb intake to 25 grams a day before they reach ketosis. This is especially true for type 2 diabetics.

If you need to decrease your carb intake to 25 grams a day, then you will need to increase your healthy fat consumption accordingly. You can increase your intake of nuts, almond butter, avocado, coconut oil, olive oil, flaxseed oil, and even add them to smoothies made with coconut milk, coconut oil, and almond butter. Consult your doctor if you have diabetes. Your blood sugar may drop dramatically on a ketogenic diet, and your medication may need to be adjusted.

> **FACTOID**
>
> The FDA maintains that MSG is GRAS (generally recognized as safe) for you to consume.[20]

GETTING A HANDLE ON *MILD* DEMENTIA

If your dementia, or the dementia of a loved one, is mild then follow the modified Mediterranean Diet carefully. The key elements to eliminate from your diet include:

- Gluten (wheat, rye, barley)
- Corn
- Fried food
- MSG
- NutraSweet
- Hydrogenated fats and trans fats
- All processed foods
- Sugar
- Limit polyunsaturated fats (corn oil, sunflower oil, safflower oil)

It comes back to inflammation again. The refined grains/corn and wheat usually cause inflammation, commonly found in those who suffer from dementia, Alzheimer's, and memory loss.

I have found two of the worst common ingredients for dementia sufferers to be MSG and NutraSweet. These are incredibly bad for the brain. Get off those as quickly as you can. MSG contains glutamic acid and NutraSweet contains aspartic acid. Both of these are neurotoxic and kill neurons by exciting them to death.

However, spotting MSG is sometimes not that easy because it can often be hidden within the ingredients. These additives are still MSG:

glutamate, monosodium glutamate, MSG, calcium caseinate, autolyzed yeast extract, hydrolyzed protein, hydrolyzed vegetable protein, hydrolyzed plant protein, yeast extract, plant protein extract, textured protein, hydrolyzed oat flour and sodium caseinate, monopotassium glutamate, glutamic acid, gelatin and Ajinomoto.[21]

I always say that if you cannot pronounce it or do not know what it is, I do not recommend that you eat it! Also, there is a raging battle behind the scenes as to the amount of MSG in processed foods that needs to be reported on the label. This means that although what you eat causes inflammation, there is supposedly no MSG because the amount per serving falls below the legal limit so a company is not required by law to list it on the label. One more reason to avoid processed foods. Practically speaking, when in doubt . . . don't!

Trans fats and hydrogenated or partially hydrogenated fats cause inflammation in the brain, and inflammation is the root cause of memory loss, dementia, and Alzheimer's disease. Anything that inflames the brain in any way must be removed from your diet. A product can be labeled zero trans fats, according to the FDA, if it contains less than 500 mg of trans fats per serving. That's why it is important to read the ingredients, and if a package lists hydrogenated or partially hydrogenated fats, then don't buy that food.

> **HEALTH TIP**
>
> The Cardiff University found that following four of these five behaviors could reduce risk of dementia by 60 percent:
>
> - Regular exercise
> - Not smoking
> - Having a low body weight
> - A healthy diet
> - Low alcohol intake

Once you get rid of the bad, it is time to pour on the good. Here are my top ten recommendations for clearing and empowering your brain:

1. Regular exercise 5 days a week for 30 minutes
2. Coconut oil
3. Fast at least twelve hours a night
4. Sleep eight hours every night
5. B12 supplements (methylcobalamin)
6. Curcumin
7. Anti-inflammatory diet
8. DHA supplements
9. Lower stress
10. Eliminate gluten

With the modified Mediterranean Diet as your foundation, which is the best anti-inflammatory diet in the world, your brain will usually begin to heal. Your brain, specifically, will begin to clear up. I have seen many dementia patients' brains "turn on" after several months on the modified Mediterranean Diet. The cloud lifts and they are back!

Candace was like that. When she and her husband came in to see me, talking to her reminded me of a light bulb that was blinking on and off. She was trying her best, but her brain was almost sputtering.

We immediately cut out the MSG, diet soda and sugar-free gum (they have NutraSweet), and gluten. No more trips with the grandkids to fast-food restaurants, that was for sure. She also jumped onto the modified Mediterranean Diet and began to exercise just fifteen minutes a day, five days a week. In both cases, her husband helped considerably.

Literally, it was just six months and her light was fully on. There was no sputtering or blinking on and off with her. She was engaged, and that meant everything to her, to her husband, and to her grandchildren.

If you or someone you love is battling dementia, Alzheimer's, or another form of dementia, there is hope! Also make sure that you do not have sleep apnea. I have found that many of my dementia patients have sleep apnea, and their brain cells are usually starving for oxygen without them even being aware of the problem. If you have early dementia or age-associated memory impairment, ask your primary care physician to order a sleep study to rule out sleep apnea. It is my intention that you be inspired, motivated, and encouraged. But I want to also challenge you to take action now.

Don't wait another day.

CHAPTER ELEVEN

R

YOUR JOURNEY

Chapter Eleven is all about getting a handle on ADHD and autism. The modified Mediterranean Diet plays a big role in finding answers for parents and caregivers of young patients with ADHD and autism. With the right diet, and eliminating the trigger foods that cause such inflammation, the results are astounding.

Don Colbert, MD

BEAT ADHD AND AUTISM
with the Modified Mediterranean Diet

YOUNG TIMMY HAD RECENTLY been diagnosed with ADHD. He was only eight years old, which was just about the normal age when children are diagnosed with ADHD.

His mother did not want to medicate her son for the foreseeable future, so her coming to my office was, she hoped, going to give her some encouragement and viable options going forward.

As we discussed cravings, the modified Mediterranean Diet, foods, menus, and other medically related details, you could almost see the weight start to lift off her shoulders. She could see a glimmer of light ahead!

She and Timmy went on the modified Mediterranean Diet, and while she lost weight, he seemed to really respond well to the change in diet. They removed gluten completely for the first year, and really worked to minimize corn and sugar, and they rotated dairy every four days. On special occasions, they would still do fast food or birthday cakes, but it was very much kept to a minimum.

Because they did the diet together, the results were better. Also, he began to see not only the logic behind making good food choices, but he was able to tell when he was slacking off.

We met several times during that first year, but when a year had passed, she was no longer worried about medications . . . because Timmy didn't need any! In school, he was becoming less and less "one of those problem children," she was pleased to say.

She was also happy about her own weight loss, but even more so, she was excited to see Timmy beginning to self-manage and take responsibility for himself.

She also quit coming to see me because she no longer needed me. That happens with about 80 percent of my patients; they get well and don't need to come back. I'm not complaining! I do recommend that they have periodic physical exams and screening tests.

For Timmy and his mother, growing up with ADHD, whether it is a proper diagnosis or not, it is certainly doable!

FOODS THAT USUALLY CONTRIBUTE TO ADHD AND AUTISM

- Artificial food coloring (primarily Red #40, Blue #2, Yellow #5 and #6)
- Food additives and preservatives
- Sugars and artificial sweeteners
- Caffeine (coffee, sodas, energy drinks)
- MSG (potato chips, frozen dinners, cold cuts, gravies, ranch dressing, salty-flavored snacks, many fast foods)
- Trans fats (margarine, cake icing, donuts, Bisquick Original)
- Gluten (wheat, rye, barley)

DEALING WITH ADHD AND AUTISM

The mental health disorder of ADHD (attention deficit hyperactivity disorder) is typically broken into three categories: inattentive (ADD), hyperactive, and impulsive. Naturally, most children diagnosed with ADHD have a combination of these three symptoms.

Approximately 11 percent of children four to seventeen years of age (6.4 million) have been diagnosed with ADHD as of 2011, so says the CDC. They paint an even darker picture when they note that things are getting even worse, for rates of ADHD diagnosis increased an average of 3 percent per year from 1997 to 2006 and an average of approximately 5 percent per year from 2003 to 2011.

It's only getting worse, and ADHD is costing American taxpayers over $40 billion per year.[22]

> **CRAVINGS**
>
> Those with ADHD or autism typically crave: *pizza.*

The overmedication or undermedication of children is a debate that will no doubt never end, but I have found that most of the children who get on the modified Mediterranean Diet and cut out wheat, corn, sugar, and processed foods, as well as rotate dairy every four days, usually have a marked improvement.

Are we curing it? In some cases, yes! In others, we are learning how to manage and control it. As I've said, the solution always has a way of coming back to our diet, and with ADHD, that is especially the case.

Autism, which has to do with early brain development, is a bit different. The abrupt improvement by getting on the modified Mediterranean Diet is still there, but it is more about managing and controlling the autism than it is about curing it. Still, being able to minimize many of the symptoms of autism is a great help and relief to parents, caregivers, and patients.

As expected, autism is also on the rise. The prevalence of autism in US children increased by 119.4 percent from 2000 (1 in 150) to 2010 (1 in 68).[23] That is a huge increase, and the Autism Society estimates annual costs in the next ten years to be $200–400 billion.

Both of these (ADHD and autism) are mental health issues that children face, and on an ever-increasing scale. As parents, relatives, or caregivers, your role is one of support and direction.

Can you do something on a practical level that will bring practical beneficial results? Yes!

Is there hope? Yes!

Can you start today? *Yes!*

REAL ANSWERS FOR ADHD AND AUTISM PATIENTS

It is because ADHD and autism are mental health issues that the modified Mediterranean Diet is so effective. It is, after all, the best anti-inflammatory diet on the planet.

I tell parents of children with ADHD or autism that we need to find the foods that scramble the brain. That's our focus. That is also why wheat and refined grains, corn, dairy, MSG, fake sugars (NutraSweet) and sugars, processed foods, and toxic fats (trans fats, fried foods, and excessive polyunsaturated fats such as corn oil, cottonseed oil, sunflower oil, safflower oil, soybean oil, etc.) are the first to go.

I have had hundreds of patients—be they suffering from autism, ADD, ADHD, dementia, Alzheimer's, memory loss, obesity, diabetes, IBS, autoimmune disease, hypertension, or acne—experience significant and sometimes immediate improvement after getting off wheat and corn, let alone the other inflammatory foods.

The fact is, with ADHD and autism patients, refined grains, wheat, corn, dairy, MSG, fake sugars and sugars, processed foods, and trans fats and fried foods are the biggest causes of inflammation. If it scrambles the brain—which it does—then it only makes sense to cut it out of their diet as quickly as possible.

That's where we begin, but each patient is different. It is about finding the foods that cause inflammation. For severe ADHD, autism, and ADD, I would suggest that they get an Alcat Test (more on Alcat Testing in Appendix D) done to help clarify the exact food sensitivities for that child.

With children, it's not all about taking foods away. We don't want to be too restrictive. They are growing and developing rapidly, so we must replace inflammatory foods with non-inflammatory foods.

For example, since we don't want the young patients losing weight, the dairy that autism patients give up can be replaced with rice milk, coconut milk, or almond milk. I would add a multivitamin with adequate amounts of B vitamins, a chewable calcium supplement, and omega-3 supplements as well as probiotics.

FOODS THAT USUALLY RELIEVE ADHD AND AUTISM

- Wild salmon, wild trout, wild sardines
- Berries (blueberries, blackberries, strawberries, raspberries)
- Vegetables (kale, spinach, broccoli, cabbage)
- Walnuts, pecans, almonds, cashews
- Hummus, beans, peas, lentils
- Avocados, olive oil
- Steel-cut oatmeal

For the ADHD patients, for example, fake sugars (such as NutraSweet and aspartame) and MSG are excitotoxins and literally excite the brain, so eliminating those are a must. Limiting sugar in general is very important for ADHD patients, but with certain foods, moderation is the key because we do not want them to lose weight (unless they are overweight or obese). You can limit or rotate their dairy and non-GMO corn every three to four days rather than eating it at every meal, and they will probably do fine. I would recommend eliminating wheat for six months and then only eating it in small amounts once or twice a week thereafter. Your child can eat gluten-free bread, brown rice, brown rice pasta, and brown rice crackers instead of wheat products.

Some of my young patients are still on Ritalin, but they are often able to reduce or come completely off of it within a few months. That is another benefit of reducing or eliminating the inflammatory foods.

THE MODIFIED MEDITERRANEAN DIET FOR ADHD AND AUTISM

How motivated are you to take action? Usually children are the ones who suffer from ADHD and autism, but as a parent or caregiver, you play an integral role. Talking about motivation is for both you and the child. It will help you tremendously to clarify your "why" for helping your child with ADHD or autism. Why do you want to do this? Why do you want to beat ADHD or autism?

Work on your answer and refine it until it's a burning, white-hot passion that drives you to do whatever it takes to be healthy. Let it propel you to where you want to go, which is a healthy lifestyle that gives you the life and freedom that you want!

Now follows the foundational modified Mediterranean Diet, except in several places you will see that it is altered slightly to best get a handle on ADHD and autism.

Level #1: fruits, vegetables, nuts, beans, and other legumes. Salads consist of dark green leafy lettuce, fresh vine-ripened tomatoes, broccoli, spinach, peppers, onions, and cucumbers. Serve vegetables in salads, as appetizers, or as a main or side dish. Fruits are usually a dessert or snack. Use nuts as toppings to add flavor and texture. The beans and legumes are usually in soups, added to salads, used as dips (i.e., hummus), or as a main dish.

Suggestions: Start with a large salad with lunch and dinner (no croutons). Eat vegetables 3 servings a day and more if able. Eat raw, steam, stir-fry, or cook under low heat with olive oil, macadamia nut oil, or coconut oil. Eat 1 to 2 servings of fruit a day (blueberries, blackberries, strawberries, raspberries, lemons, limes, or any other types of fruit, but avoid fruit juice).

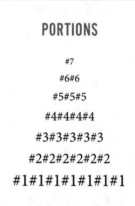

PORTIONS

#7
#6#6
#5#5#5
#4#4#4#4
#3#3#3#3#3
#2#2#2#2#2#2
#1#1#1#1#1#1#1#1

Suggestions: Eat ½–2 cups daily of beans, bean soups, peas, legumes, lentils, and hummus, preferably before meals.

Level #2: steel-cut oats and quinoa, millet or millet bread, brown rice, brown rice pasta, brown rice bread, and sweet potatoes. If you are not gluten sensitive, trying to lose weight, or suffering from high blood pressure, diabetes, or high cholesterol, then potatoes, sprouted bread (i.e., Ezekiel 4:9 bread), or fermented bread (i.e., sourdough bread) are fine on occasion and with moderation, such as every three to four days.

Altered: For autism, eliminate gluten (wheat, barley, rye), corn, and white rice completely from your diet. After six months, rotating grains and corn every four days may be acceptable for patients with ADHD and for some with autism, but the corn should be non-GMO.

Level #3: olive oil, used instead of other oils, margarine, etc. Not only for cooking, it is commonly mixed with balsamic vinegar as a salad dressing. Small amounts of organic butter are fine.

> *Altered:* Eliminate all fried foods, hydrogenated oils, and trans fats completely from your diet. Limit polyunsaturated fats (corn oil, sunflower oil, safflower oil, soybean oil, and avoid GMO oils such as most canola oil and cottonseed oil).

> *Suggestions:* Consume 2 to 4 tablespoons of extra-virgin olive oil daily, with cooking and on salads (with balsamic vinegar or any other type of vinegar).

> *Suggestions:* Eat one handful of raw nuts (almonds, hazelnuts, pecans, cashews, walnuts, macadamia) daily.

Level #4: cheese and yogurt, in small amounts. Freshly grated Parmesan on pasta or a little feta cheese on a salad is common. Yogurt (about a cup a day) is how milk is usually eaten, and it is low fat or nonfat, served with fresh fruit added. Yogurt is also a salad dressing (i.e., mixed with dill, garlic, onion, and cucumbers).

> *Altered:* With autism, eliminate dairy. With ADHD, rotate dairy every four days in limited amounts, such as 4 to 8 ounces of milk or yogurt or a small amount of cheese.

Level #5: fish, eaten more than other meats, in about 4-ounce portions several times a week.

> **Altered:** Eat the lowest mercury fish possible. (See Appendix C for list of fish.)

Level #6: chicken, turkey, and eggs. Chicken in 3- to 6-ounce portions a few times a week is common. The meat is usually skinless and added to soups, stews, and other dishes loaded with vegetables. Only 1 to 6 eggs per week with 1 egg yolk/3 egg white ratio.

Level #7: red meat, in the form of beef, veal, pork, sheep, lamb, and goats, is eaten only a few times a month. It is then often served as a topping to a vegetable, pasta, or rice dish. Avoid or limit red meat to 3 to 6 ounces once or twice a week.

> **Suggestions:** Rotate vegetables and meats every 4 days (do not eat the same foods every day). For example, day 1, eat chicken; day 2, turkey; day 3, salmon; and so on.

REAL HELP FOR ADHD AND AUTISM

I cannot tell you how many children have come through my office doors needing help with their ADHD, ADD, or autism. My heart goes out to them and their parents, and I do all I can to help.

Usually, the marked improvement from being on the modified Mediterranean Diet and eliminating certain foods from their diet is such a radical and positive step forward that they are super appreciative. Many times, it was just one or two things that we adjusted that brought healing.

Do we cure the child? Sometimes we do, but often their improvement is more like a big step forward toward successful control and management. It's learning to live with it, but to the best degree possible!

Young Carl had ADD when I saw him and his parents. We looked at food from a moderation or rotation point of view rather than from an elimination point of view. That was more their style as a family, and though I thought elimination of wheat, corn, and sugar would have brought about quicker results, they were willing to slowly change the family's eating habits. They would wean Carl off certain foods, but slowly.

This meant more foods prepared in their home rather than eating out, and they ate a lot more fruits, vegetables, salads, and homemade soups, and a lot less processed foods. The craving for pizza was satisfied with the occasional homemade pizza made from gluten-free flour rather than pizza from a fast-food restaurant. They introduced most of the modified Mediterranean Diet to their family over the months that followed.

The shift took time, but a year later they were very pleased with the results. Carl was performing better in school, he was off his Ritalin medication, and he was able to pay much better attention to tasks.

They also decided they only needed to see me once a year, which happens all the time! I'm used to that.

The most important thing was that their son was on his way to a better life with his better health.

CHAPTER TWELVE

℞

YOUR JOURNEY

Chapter Twelve is all about the battle with mental illness. Learn how to fight at both levels—the mental level and the diet level—for it is a dual approach to beating mental illness. You can overcome! So many patients have had amazing results when they bring the brain and the body into balance. You can too!

Don Colbert, MD

BEAT MENTAL ILLNESS
with the Modified Mediterranean Diet

I GREW UP WITH SOCIAL PHOBIA, though at the time I had no idea it was a phobia. I was picked on when I was younger by my older sister, which helped program me to think that I was ugly and inferior, but that only masked my social phobia.

When I would walk into a room, I felt panicky and thought that everyone was looking at me and judging me. My pulse would quicken and I would break out in a cold sweat. As a medical student, I never raised my hand to ask a question. Anything to draw attention to myself was usually avoided.

As a medical doctor, I found myself speaking more in public and giving advice to a lot of people. I was not necessarily afraid of public speaking, which is the number one phobia; in my case it was the social phobia of when I walked in the doors (when everyone was looking at me) until the point where I was actually talking.

One friend, who was a pastor, would have me occasionally come and speak to his growing audience about health, nutrition, dieting, and more. But before he called me up on stage, I would be sitting there sweating like a burger on a grill. It was too much for me. My heart was racing and my breathing was shallow. He kept asking me to speak, and I kept agreeing to do it, and eventually I was able to overcome the social phobia.

I thought something was wrong with me, but it wasn't until years later that I learned I had social phobia. According to the ADAA (Anxiety and Depression Association of America), I am not alone. Such disorders are very common,[24] affecting countless people every single day:

- Specific phobias: 8.7 percent of US population
- Social anxiety disorder: 6.8 percent
- Major depressive disorder: 6.7 percent (between ages 15–44)
- Post-traumatic stress disorder: 3.5 percent
- Generalized anxiety disorder: 3.1 percent
- Panic disorder: 2.7 percent
- Persistent depressive disorder: 1.5 percent
- Obsessive-compulsive disorder: 1 percent

I used to suffer from social phobia, but now I can go into a room and don't even get nervous. I've reprogrammed distortional thinking and dealt with the lies. I've learned that phobias can usually be overcome with a mixture of a simple five-minute phobia cure, reprogramming distortional thinking with cognitive behavioral therapy, trauma resolution therapy, and diet.

CONFRONTING MENTAL ILLNESS

How do we get mental illness anyway?

Some mental illness is inherited, some is programmed into us by learning distortional thought patterns from dysfunctional family members, and some is triggered by emotional or physical trauma, but that is certainly not an epidemic or an illness. Sometimes there are outside triggers that can lead to mental illness. I have seen too many patients who smoked marijuana when they were teenagers, and now they are bipolar or schizophrenic, to not see the connection. Marijuana can, figuratively speaking, flip a switch in some people, and mental illness is a direct result. Marijuana also diminishes passions and creates lethargy, and I would say that marijuana dumbs people down and turns many into slugs, and that is no help for mental health patients.

> **CRAVINGS**
>
> Those with mental issues typically crave: *sugars, breads, and dairy.*

But head trauma and marijuana are not the leading causes of mental illness. According to the Mayo Clinic, mental illnesses in general are thought to be caused by various genetic and environmental factors such as:

- *Inherited traits*: Mental illness is more common in people whose biological (blood) relatives also have a mental illness. Certain genes may increase your risk of developing a mental illness, and your life situation may trigger it.
- *Environmental exposures before birth*: Exposure to viruses, toxins, alcohol, or drugs while in the womb can sometimes be linked to mental illness.
- *Brain chemistry*: Biochemical changes in the brain are thought to affect mood and other aspects of mental health. Naturally occurring brain chemicals called neurotransmitters play a role in some mental illnesses. In some cases, hormonal imbalances affect mental health.

Of all the mental disorders, anxiety disorders (including PTSD, OCD, and specific phobias) collectively rank at the top as the mental disorder that affects most Americans.[25] And as you might expect, nearly half of those diagnosed with anxiety are also diagnosed with depression.[26]

Depression is one of the most common types of mental illness, affecting more than 26 percent of the US adult population.[27] It is estimated that by 2020, depression will be the second leading cause of disability throughout the world, trailing only coronary artery disease.[28]

Not surprisingly, evidence has shown that mental disorders, especially depressive disorders, are strongly related to chronic diseases like diabetes, cancer, cardiovascular disease, asthma, and obesity.[29] The CDC adds that mental disorders also lead to physical inactivity, smoking, excessive drinking, and insufficient sleep, which makes the problems only worse for patients.

Not good news at all.

> ### FOODS THAT MAY INCREASE ANXIETY
>
> - Coffee, caffeinated drinks, energy drinks
> - Smoothies, fruit juice
> - Alcohol
> - MSG
> - Candy, sodas, cookies
> - Artificial sweeteners (diet sodas, chewing gum)
> - Gluten (wheat, rye, barley)

BATTLING MENTAL ILLNESS

If you are reading this chapter, perhaps you or someone you know is battling mental illness. I recognize that this can be a tough road . . . but it is something you can beat.

I believe you have the ability to choose healing and health. You can walk free. Yes, it requires good choices, effort, and changes, but you can do it. You are not bound by genetics, environment, or chemistry.

I have seen some incredible cases, with patients who seem to be beyond all help and all hope, yet they have overcome. It is possible. I've seen it too many times to doubt anyone's ability to overcome.

Sure, the statistics are doom and gloom, but the battle for your mental wellness is fought on two fronts:

#1 battle: in your mind
#2 battle: in your diet

FOODS THAT HELP DECREASE ANXIETY

- Tryptophan-rich foods (turkey, chicken, bananas)
- Wild salmon, wild trout, wild sardines
- Brown rice, brown rice pasta, brown rice bread, millet bread
- Beans, peas, lentils, hummus
- Sweet potatoes, steel-cut oatmeal
- Walnuts, almonds, cashews
- Kale, spinach, other leafy greens

Mental illness, because of its very nature, is a battle that must be fought in your mind, and because your diet affects every area of your body and your life, it is also a battle in your diet.

So where should you begin? For the short term, medication may play an important and helpful role. The medications that treat mental illness are powerful and very useful, but I believe for many they are ideally suited for the short term and not a lifetime. For the long term, that is where a healthy diet and healthy lifestyle come into play. Treating the symptoms is great for the moment, but unless you get to the core of the issue, nothing truly has changed. Please do not stop taking your medication, but as your condition improves, your medical doctor or psychiatrist may eventually be able to wean you down or wean you off your medication.

Next, I suggest that you strategically address both the mental and the dietary side of things at the same time. You certainly want to walk free, but it's more of a marathon than a sprint.

#1 Battle: In Your Mind

The battle of the mind requires a change in your thinking. I have found that deep down, at the very root of mental illness, is some "stinkin' thinkin'" that needs to be set right.

That may sound very general and nonchalant, and I'm not making light of any mental illness at all, but it is nonetheless true. Somewhere, in the past, a lie or trauma usually takes root in your heart and mind that is today wreaking havoc in your very soul. It must be pulled out, like a weed, and replaced with the truth. Proverbs 4:23 clearly states, "Keep your heart with all diligence, for out of it spring the issues of life."

Attitude formation is key to setting your mind on the proper track. The author of *Know Love, Live Loved* explains very clearly just how attitudes are formed.[30] There are three basic steps to forming an attitude:

Step #1—*Input*: Everything since birth is used by your subconscious mind as input from which attitudes are formed. When you are older and realize the need to change your attitudes, you obviously can't start over at birth. What you can do, however, is to change the input. This has a way of positively affecting your mind and your entire body.

Step #2—*Processing of inputs*: As you have heard what other people said to you and observed what they did in their own lives, you processed that information and chose your attitudes. As you acted on your chosen belief, it gradually became established as a habit of thought—an attitude.

Step #3—*Reinforcement*: When you make a tentative choice of an attitude, it eventually becomes firmly entrenched by reinforcement as you follow it day after day. There is nothing mystical about it. It simply happens.

FOODS THAT USUALLY CONTRIBUTE TO DEPRESSION

- Gluten (wheat, rye, barley)
- Refined processed grains, white rice, processed corn (popcorn, corn chips, corn tortillas)
- Sugar, artificial sweeteners
- Alcohol (beer, wine, spirits)
- Polyunsaturated fats (sunflower oil, safflower oil, cottonseed oil, corn oil)
- Trans fats (shortening, donuts, margarine), fried foods
- MSG

This is where things get powerful. When you become aware that some specific attitude is holding you back in some way, you can change that attitude.

Changing a habit of action or thought is not simple or necessarily quick, but it is certainly possible. You must first make a conscious choice to change! Breaking the old cycle of habit formation is the key to changing your attitudes. The following principle shows exactly how it works:

Sow a thought, reap an action.
Sow an action, reap a habit.
Sow a habit, reap character.
Sow character, reap a destiny.

As you work to change your attitude, remember that attitudes operate on three levels: thought, speech, and behavior. What you fill your mind with is eventually translated into the words you speak, and then your words are put into action. If you are not pleased with your results, you can intervene in the process of attitude formation by focusing on what you think, say, or do.

If you want to change your attitude, you must change the way you think. You must be aware of what goes on in your head, however, before you can change it. Whenever you catch yourself thinking a lie that feeds your mental illness, stop and tell yourself the truth. The important thing to do is to break the automatic negative thought pattern. It will take some time, so keep at it.

Intervening at the point of thoughts is often the easiest place at which you can begin to make a change. Second Corinthians 10:4–5 makes it plain when it says, "For the weapons of our warfare are not carnal but mighty in God for pulling down strongholds, casting down arguments and every high thing that exalts itself against the knowledge of God, bringing every thought into captivity to the obedience of Christ."

Then listen to yourself as you talk. How often do you use negative words? How often do you express doubt that you will break free? Write out some positive words to use the next time the chance arises. Be sure these words express the attitude you want to adopt. Practice long enough so that you will remember the positive words when you need them.

Where you intervene is up to you, since your personality is unique and your abilities are different. Attitudes, because they are habits of thought, do not happen overnight. You will not change them with one attempt, so be patient and give yourself time to absorb enough new, positive input to make the desired change.

Finally, what you must have in your heart and mind is an I-will-not-be-denied attitude that pursues your health no matter what! This brings in the willingness to press through any area of need, be it forgiveness therapy, phobia therapy, trauma resolution therapy, cognitive behavioral therapy, asking for help, you name it. When you are tenacious and refuse to let go, that is when you get what you want.

FOODS THAT MAY RELIEVE DEPRESSION

- Dark chocolate low in sugar
- Green tea
- Berries (blueberries, blackberries, strawberries, raspberries)
- Wild salmon, wild trout, wild sardines
- High-tryptophan foods (turkey, chicken, bananas)

This is precisely in line with Matthew 7:7–8 as it explains, "Keep on asking and it will be given you; keep on seeking and you will find; keep on knocking [reverently] and [the door] will be opened to you. For everyone who keeps on asking receives; and he who keeps on seeking finds; and to him who keeps on knocking, [the door] will be opened" (AMP).

There is help and there is hope. And your mental health is worth it!

#2 Battle: In Your Diet

In the battle of your diet, it also is going to require a change. With mental illness, I have seen many patients who crave foods that inflame the brain, which usually fuels the mental illness.

To correct that, we begin with the modified Mediterranean Diet. I also add some supplements because many times mental health patients have specific needs. We may run some special tests to gain further insight into their needs.

However, gluten is one item that I immediately remove from their diet. Sometimes dairy, but always gluten.

The goal is to get the body (GI tract) and brain balanced and healthy. That always positively affects the mind.

THE MODIFIED MEDITERRANEAN DIET FOR DEPRESSION, ANXIETY, BIPOLAR DISORDER, AND SCHIZOPHRENIA

How motivated are you to take action? It will help you tremendously to clarify your "why" for getting healthy and whole. Why do you want to do this? Why do you want to beat your mental illness?

Work on your answer and refine it until it's a burning, white-hot passion that drives you to do whatever it takes to be healthy. Let it propel you to where you want to go, which is a healthy lifestyle that gives you the life and freedom that you want!

Now follows the foundational modified Mediterranean Diet, except in several places you will see that it is altered slightly to best get a handle on mental illness.

Level #1: fruits, vegetables, nuts, beans, and other legumes. Salads consist of dark green leafy lettuce, fresh vine-ripened tomatoes, broccoli, spinach, peppers, onions, and cucumbers. Serve vegetables in salads, as appetizers, or as a main or side dish. Fruits are usually a dessert or snack. Use nuts as toppings to add flavor and texture. The beans and legumes are usually in soups, added to salads, used as dips (i.e., hummus), or as a main dish.

Suggestions: Start with a large salad with lunch and dinner (no croutons). Eat vegetables 3 servings a day and more if able. Eat raw, steam, stir-fry, or cook under low heat with olive oil, macadamia nut oil, or coconut oil. Eat 1 to 2 servings of fruit a day (blueberries, blackberries, strawberries, raspberries, lemons, limes ,or any other types of fruit, but avoid fruit juice).

Suggestions: Eat ½ to 2 cups daily of beans, bean soups, peas, lentils, legumes, and hummus, preferably before meals.

Level #2: steel-cut oats and quinoa, millet or millet bread, brown rice, and sweet potatoes. If you are not gluten sensitive, trying to lose weight, or suffering from high blood pressure, diabetes, or high cholesterol, then potatoes, sprouted bread (i.e., Ezekiel 4:9 bread), or fermented bread (i.e., sourdough bread) are fine on occasion and with moderation.

Altered: Eliminate gluten (wheat, barley, and rye), corn, rice, and wheat pasta completely from your diet (see Appendix F for list of foods containing gluten). You may eat brown rice, brown rice bread, and brown rice pasta.

Level #3: olive oil, used instead of other oils, margarine, etc. Not only for cooking, it is commonly mixed with balsamic vinegar as a salad dressing. Small amounts of organic butter are fine.

Altered: Eliminate all fried foods completely from your diet, as well as trans fats and hydrogenated fats, and limit polyunsaturated fats (corn oil, cotton seed oil, sunflower oil, safflower oil, and soybean oil) to a very small amount. Avoid GMO canola oil.

Suggestions: Consume 2 to 4 tablespoons of extra-virgin olive oil daily, with cooking and on salads (with balsamic vinegar or any other type of vinegar).

Suggestions: Eat one handful of raw nuts (almonds, hazelnuts, pecans, cashews, walnuts, macadamia) daily.

Level #4: cheese and yogurt, in small amounts. Freshly grated Parmesan on pasta or a little feta cheese on a salad is common. Yogurt (about a cup a day) is how milk is usually eaten, and it is low fat or nonfat, served with fresh fruit added. Yogurt is also a salad dressing (i.e., mixed with dill, garlic, onion, and cucumbers).

Altered: You need to eliminate dairy if you have schizophrenia or bipolar disease. At minimum, rotate dairy every 4 days, 4 to 8 ounces of skim milk or low-fat, low-sugar yogurt and small amounts of cheese.

Level #5: fish, eaten more than other meats, in about 4- to 6-ounce portions several times a week.

Altered: Eat the lowest mercury fish possible. Choose wild salmon on a regular basis (see Appendix C for list of fish).

Level #6: chicken, turkey, and eggs. Chicken in 3- to 6-ounce portions a few times a week is common. The meat is usually skinless and added to soups, stews, and other dishes loaded with vegetables. Only 1 to 6 eggs per week with 1 egg yolk/3 egg white ratio.

Level #7: red meat, in the form of beef, veal, pork, sheep, lamb, and goats, is eaten only a few times a month (at most, 3- to 6-ounce portions once or twice a week). It is then often served as a topping to a vegetable, pasta, or rice dish.

Suggestions: Rotate vegetables and meats every 4 days (do not eat the same foods every day). For example, day 1, eat chicken; day 2, turkey; day 3, salmon; and so on.

With mental illness, it is very important to eliminate MSG and NutraSweet, which are excitotoxins. One should also avoid or limit sugar and processed foods. Trans fats and fried foods should be avoided, and one should limit polyunsaturated fats.

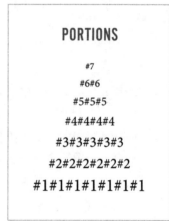

PORTIONS

#7
#6#6
#5#5#5
#4#4#4#4
#3#3#3#3#3
#2#2#2#2#2#2
#1#1#1#1#1#1#1

BEATING MENTAL ILLNESS

Can you beat mental illness? I have seen it beat many times, so the answer is a resounding "yes!"

Sean Miller is a great example (that is his real name). When he came to see me, he would have labeled himself a real "basket case."

He had been in and out of hospitals, placed on suicide watch, was on a lot of medications, and was labeled as suffering from psychosis, OCD, schizophrenia, and depression.

His family did have some mental health issues, but he was very popular and healthy while in school. Nothing seemed amiss. At age twenty-three, he began to experience troubling thoughts, then voices, and then those voices began to threaten him if he didn't comply.

The tormenting voices and demands and sudden mood swings to compensate for the irrational behavior had almost ruined his life. He had lost friends, couldn't be employed, his marriage was on the rocks, and his health was deteriorating. He couldn't sleep well and he looked pale and ashen. He went through spells of intense anxiety and then extreme guilt.

The voices would tell him that if he flew on a plane that he would die or that if he went to the bank he would die. A simple task, like going grocery shopping, was riddled with decisions and voices and demands. The panic attacks were constant and the more he listened to the voices, the more the voices seemed real.

"I couldn't find peace of mind," he says. "And any nightmares were a break from the daily nonstop battle."

He lost joy in everything he once enjoyed. Life felt flat and meaningless.

Interestingly, he initially did not seek help because he didn't know what was happening, but as his symptoms worsened, he finally reached the point where he needed to be hospitalized. His stays were as short as a week to as long as three months.

The side effects of the medication were not good. "I did not want this to be my norm," he explained. "I wanted to beat this thing and to move on with life."

He tried going off the medications, but that only made things worse. In fact, at one point he went delusional and his wife had to call the police. He was taken away in handcuffs. He was losing the ability to see himself doing things; he was losing his sense of connection to the world, and that produced a whole new wave of terror.

His wife came to the conclusion that the medications would never be able to heal Sean. There was no pill that would fix him. Their doctors had only said, "Get used to living this way for the rest of your life." But they needed more than something to treat the symptoms. They wanted to live again!

In late 2006, somehow she found one of my books and called my office to set up an appointment. Sean was deathly afraid of flying to see me, but his wife coaxed him into coming. His psychiatrist also double-medicated him, but it was still touch-and-go until the plane took off.

When the plane arrived safely, he realized he was alive

FOODS THAT USUALLY WORSEN SCHIZOPHRENIA

- All gluten (wheat, rye, barley)
- MSG
- Artificial sweeteners
- Alcohol (beer, wine, spirits)
- Caffeinated drinks, energy drinks
- Sugar, refined carbohydrates
- Trans fats/fried foods

. . . and that the voices were lying. He didn't die on the way as the voices had promised. His doubt that the voices were real was a breakthrough for him, which was part of his ongoing mental battle.

When we met, I explained that what he was suffering from was treatable and that when we were done, it would be as if he had never had a problem.

They could barely believe me, but they were both ravenously

hungry to find help, hope, and answers. They were determined, and I was glad to help.

We began with the modified Mediterranean Diet, the best anti-inflammatory diet out there. I immediately recommended that we get him off gluten and dairy. I also put him on some healthy oils for the brain, some DHA supplements, and some natural supplements to help him sleep, along with an exercise program to get his muscles and energy level back up. All of it was designed to get his brain balanced. I also had him take a neurotransmitter test, and the results helped us refine our dietary efforts and supplement regimen.

FOODS THAT MAY IMPROVE SCHIZOPHRENIA

- Omega-3 oils (wild sardines, wild herring, wild salmon, wild trout)
- Walnuts, pecans, almonds, cashews
- Berries (blueberries, blackberries, strawberries, raspberries)
- Flax seeds, flax seed oil, chia seeds, salba seeds
- Beans, peas, lentils, hummus
- High-tryptophan foods (turkey, chicken, bananas)
- Brown rice, brown rice pasta, brown rice bread

Mental illness, like any sickness, is far more than just treating symptoms. There is a strong connection between good health in your gut and good health in your brain. The foods that used to cause inflammation in his brain, such as gluten, pasta, and dairy, were removed from Sean's diet . . . and his body responded beautifully!

Four months later, Sean realized the voices were quieter. His sinus issues cleared up. What's more, his doctor was able to slowly wean him off the medications he had been taking for years.

It was like a switch was flipped, but this time it was a good one! His doctor was amazed, but Sean and his wife were beyond grateful. The more his brain and body balanced out and his health improved, the more his mental illness subsided.

Hope blossomed! Completely off all psychotic medication, Sean and his wife had the joy of facing life together, without mental illness in the picture. It was an amazing thing to witness.

> **FACTOID**
>
> Gluten is a very common inflammatory food for those with mental illness. Avoid it at all costs.

His wife so powerfully stated, "It has been a long road, but I did not think God would leave us in this dark place. I'm really glad I stayed. The recovery has been beyond what I hoped for. He's better than the man I married. There was a broken piece in him that has now healed as well. We are excited about our future ahead of us."

Today, Sean is fully recovered. He avoids gluten and dairy, and stays on the modified Mediterranean Diet. Yes, the genetic component may be there, but he can stay in remission forever.

The future—*their* future—is bright.

Your future is just as bright.

Seeing people get their lives back is what this is all about. Rest assured, no matter your ailment, there is hope!

CONCLUSION

AFTER THIRTY YEARS of practicing medicine and fervently looking for answers to my patients' core health issues, the best advice I can give anyone is that they pursue a diet and lifestyle that provides them with good health, sickness prevention, and the ability to treat actual diseases!

The only diet I have found that actually does all this is the modified Mediterranean Diet. It is truly the key to the kingdom of health.

I'm not cocky . . . I'm confident. For me and my patients, what you have read in these pages are the keys to a healthy lifestyle that cannot be beat. It's proven and it works.

If you do have one of the diseases mentioned in this book, then you have in your hands the very tools that will help you treat (cure, control, or manage) what ails you. And we are not talking about treating just the symptoms; we are talking about treating the real issues, and I love that as a medical doctor.

That Hippocratic Oath, which all medical doctors swear to uphold, states, "I will prevent disease whenever I can, for prevention is preferable to cure." Of course prevention is better, and that is why the modified Mediterranean Diet is the answer to a long-term lifestyle of health and wellness.

Remember, it was also Hippocrates who said, "Let food be thy medicine and medicine be thy food." We are doing just that! This book is *the* answer to a healthy lifestyle that is also all about prevention. Truly amazing!

I'm so confident that this healthy lifestyle is effective at treating any chronic disease that I welcome you to contact my office with what ails you. Together we can come up with a plan of attack that you can live with!

> **THOUGHT**
>
> Imagine how better our health would be if restaurants across the nation offered meals that fit the modified Mediterranean Diet!

Finally, my parting comment is one of hope. I know, when I was a patient myself, just how important hope was. Without it, we cannot face tomorrow . . . but with it, we can take on the world!

I want to leave you with hope—a hope that helps you face another tomorrow, hope to grab hold of what you want and not let go, and hope to regain or improve your health.

You can do it!

APPENDIXES

There are countless details, clauses, statistics, recommendations, and graphs that could be listed, but I'm more concerned with providing you with helpful information along your journey toward health. What follows is just that. It is brief and to the point. If you need more information, then contact my office.

Don Colbert, MD

Appendix A

MENUS FOR FOUR DAYS OF ROTATION

These suggested meals, ideally rotated every four days, follow the modified Mediterranean Diet and are intended to give you a practical starting point for your own menus, schedules, and health plans.

DAY #1

BREAKFAST (6 A.M.):
- Large bowl of steel-cut oatmeal cooked with ¼ cup berries
- Handful of walnuts (approximately 5–10)
- 1 cup of green tea or coffee, sweetened with stevia, coconut milk for creamer
- Smoothie (8 oz.) with plain coconut or almond milk, ½ frozen banana, ¼ cup frozen blueberries, raspberries, strawberries, or blackberries, 1–2 tbsp. ground flaxseeds, 1 scoop plant protein powder (may add ice or stevia to sweeten), 1 tbsp. cashew nut butter

MID-MORNING SNACK (9 A.M.):
- Granny Smith apple

LUNCH (12 P.M.):
- Large salad with extra-virgin olive oil and vinegar, with as many veggies as desired (but no croutons)

- Grilled skinless chicken breast (3–4 oz. for women, 3–6 oz. for men)
- ½ to 1 cup of black bean soup
- Steamed vegetables (as much as desired) seasoned with small amount of salt, if desired
- 1 cup of green tea, water, sparkling water, or unsweetened iced tea with lemon or lime

MID-AFTERNOON SNACK (3 P.M.):
- Handful of walnuts

DINNER (6 P.M.):
- Large salad made of romaine lettuce or other salad greens, sliced cucumber, chopped tomato, and extra-virgin olive oil and balsamic vinegar as dressing (no croutons)
- Extra-lean beef (96/4) seasoned with salt or pepper, if desired (3–4 oz. for women, 3–6 oz. for men)
- Steamed broccoli (as much as desired) seasoned with small amount of salt, if desired
- ½ to 1 cup of of broth-based vegetable or bean soup (optional) with no potatoes or pasta
- 1 cup of green tea, water, sparkling water, or unsweetened iced tea with lemon or lime

EVENING SNACK (9 P.M.):
- Lettuce wrap with chicken, onions, garlic, and other vegetables, seasoned to taste (may add a few slices of avocado)

DAY #2

BREAKFAST (6 A.M.):

- 2–3 eggs (1 yolk, 3 whites) scrambled, poached, or fried (may add onions, mushrooms, and avocado, cooked in olive oil or a small amount of organic butter if you like)
- Hash browns or sweet potato hash browns (½ cup for women, 1 cup for men) with diced onions and cooked under low heat with olive oil.
- ¼–½ cup of fruit
- 1 cup of green tea or coffee, sweetened with stevia, coconut milk for creamer

MID-MORNING SNACK (9 A.M.):

- Pear

LUNCH (12 P.M.):

- Grilled flounder (3–4 oz. for women, 3–6 oz. for men)
- Steamed asparagus (as much as desired) seasoned with lemon pepper, if desired
- ½ cup of red beans
- Large salad with plenty of colorful vegetables and extra-virgin olive oil and balsamic vinegar as dressing
- 1 cup of green tea, water, sparkling water, or unsweetened iced tea with lemon or lime

MID-AFTERNOON SNACK (3 P.M.):

- Handful of macadamia nuts

DINNER (6 P.M.):

- Large salad with plenty of colorful vegetables and extra-virgin olive oil and balsamic vinegar as dressing (no croutons)
- Bowl of broth-based vegetable soup or a bowl of lentil soup
- Grilled wild tilapia (3–4 oz. for women, 3–6 oz. for men)
- As many green vegetables as you like (broccoli, asparagus, green beans, etc.) seasoned with garlic, lemon pepper, or small amount of salt, if desired
- 1 cup of green tea, water, sparkling water, or unsweetened iced tea with lemon or lime

EVENING SNACK (9 P.M.):

- Salad with pecans and raspberries with olive oil/vinegar dressing

DAY #3

BREAKFAST (6 A.M.):
- ¾ cup gluten-free, high-fiber ceral such as Barbara's Puffins cinnamon cereal with 8 oz. coconut, almond, or skim milk and ¼ cup blueberries
- 2–3 oz. turkey bacon or turkey sausage (squeeze between two napkins to remove fat)
- 1 cup of green tea or coffee, sweetened with stevia, coconut milk for creamer

MID-MORNING SNACK (9 A.M.):
- Tangerine

LUNCH (12 P.M.):
- ½–1 cup of lima beans
- Large salad with plenty of colorful vegetables and extra-virgin olive oil and balsamic vinegar as dressing (no croutons)
- Tuna sandwich: 3–6 oz. tongol tuna topped with 1 tbsp. Smart Balance Light Mayonnaise, sliced tomato, and romaine lettuce on 1–2 slices brown rice bread, or gluten-free bread
- 1 cup of green tea, water, sparkling water, or unsweetened iced tea with lemon or lime

MID-AFTERNOON SNACK (3 P.M.):
- Handful of pecans

DINNER (6 P.M.):

- 3–6 oz. of turkey breast
- Green beans, broccoli, or other green vegetable (as much as desired) seasoned with lemon pepper, garlic, or small amount of salt, if desired
- Large salad with plenty of colorful vegetables and extra-virgin olive oil and balsamic vinegar as dressing (no croutons)
- ½-1 cup pinto beans or bean soup
- 1 cup of green tea, water, sparkling water, or unsweetened iced tea with lemon or lime

EVENING SNACK (9 P.M.):

- Bowl of broth-based vegetable soup

DAY #4

BREAKFAST (6 A.M.):

- 2 slices of gluten-free French toast (my favorite bread is Canyon Bakehouse); mix together ¼ tsp. cinnamon, ¼ tsp. vanilla extract, 2-3 egg whites and 1 yolk and dip both sides of bread in batter; cook in skillet; top with ¼–½ cup berries (blackberries, strawberries, raspberries, blueberries) sautéed in 1–2 pats of organic butter
- [Optional] 2 gluten-free pancakes topped with sautéed berries, as above
- Smoothie (8 oz.) with coconut or almond milk, ½ frozen banana or 1 tbsp. almond butter, ¼ cup frozen blueberries or raspberries, 1–2 tbsp. ground flaxseeds, 1 scoop plant protein powder (may add ice or stevia to taste)
- 1 cup of green tea or coffee, sweetened with stevia, coconut milk for creamer

MID-MORNING SNACK (9 A.M.):

- ¼ cup strawberries

LUNCH (12 P.M.):

- Large salad with plenty of colorful vegetables and extra-virgin olive oil and balsamic vinegar as dressing (no croutons)
- Grilled wild salmon (3–4 oz. for women, 3–6 oz. for men)
- Baked sweet potato (size of 1 tennis ball for women, 1–2 tennis ball size for men) with 1 tsp. of organic butter
- 1 cup of green tea, water, sparkling water, or unsweetened iced tea with lemon or lime

MID-AFTERNOON SNACK (3 P.M.):

- Handful of cashews

DINNER (6 P.M.):

- Hummus (½ cup) with 1-2 slices of gluten-free pita bread
- Large salad with plenty of colorful vegetables and extra-virgin olive oil and balsamic vinegar as dressing (no croutons)
- Grilled chicken (3–6 oz. for women, 3–6 oz. for men)
- Coleslaw (1 cup): shred half a head of cabbage and mix with 1–2 tbsp. Smart Balance Light Mayonnaise, ½ cup apple cider vinegar, 1 tbsp. celery seed, and 1 grated carrot
- Bowl of broth-based vegetable soup
- Steamed broccoli (as much as desired)
- 1 cup of green tea, water, sparkling water, or unsweetened iced tea with lemon or lime

EVENING SNACK (9 P.M.):

- Hummus (½ cup) with celery sticks

Appendix B

PESTICIDES IN FRUITS AND VEGETABLES

The amount of pesticides in fruits and vegetables depends on several factors, including the type of plant, how it grows, its skin, how it's watered, and length of growing season. According to the Environmental Working Group (EWP), there is a "Dirty Dozen" of fruits/vegetables with higher amounts of pesticides and a "Clean Fifteen" of fruits/vegetables with lesser amounts of pesticides.

The Dirty Dozen:
1. Apples
2. Peaches
3. Nectarines
4. Strawberries
5. Grapes
6. Celery
7. Spinach
8. Sweet bell peppers
9. Cucumbers
10. Cherry tomatoes
11. Snap peas (imported)
12. Potatoes

The Clean Fifteen:
1. Avocados
2. Sweet corn
3. Pineapples
4. Cabbage
5. Sweet peas (frozen)
6. Onions
7. Asparagus
8. Mangos
9. Papayas
10. Kiwi
11. Eggplant
12. Grapefruit
13. Cantaloupe
14. Cauliflower
15. Sweet potatoes

Appendix C

MERCURY-IN-FISH LIST

The amount of mercury in fish depends on factors such as the type of fish, what it eats, and where it lives. According to the Natural Resources Defense Council, this is their recommendation for eating fish:

- **Fish with least mercury** *(eat freely)*: anchovies, butterfish, catfish, clams, crab (domestic), crawfish/crayfish, croaker (Atlantic), flounder, haddock (Atlantic), hake, herring, mackerel (N. Atlantic, chub), mullet, oyster, perch (ocean), plaice, pollock, salmon (canned or fresh), sardine, scallop, shad (American), shrimp, sole (Pacific), squid (calamari), tilapia, trout (freshwater), whitefish, and whiting
- **Fish with moderate mercury** *(eat 6 servings or less per month)*: bass (striped, black), carp, cod (Alaskan), croaker (white, Pacific), halibut (Atlantic, Pacific), jacksmelt, silverside, lobster, mahi mahi, monkfish, perch (freshwater), sablefish, skate, snapper, tuna (canned chunk light, skipjack), and weakfish (sea trout)
- **Fish with high mercury** *(eat 3 servings or less per month)*: bluefish, grouper, mackerel (Spanish, Gulf), sea bass (Chilean), and tuna (canned albacore, yellow fin)
- **Fish with highest mercury** *(avoid eating)*: mackerel (king), marlin, orange roughy, shark, swordfish, tilefish, and tuna (bigeye, ahi)

Appendix D

ALCAT TESTING

I have used the Alcat Test with many patients who need greater clarification as to what foods their bodies react to and why. The test measures the non-IGE mediated reactions to foods, chemicals, and other substances. According to Alcat:

> The Alcat Test is a lab based immune stimulation test in which a patient's WBC's are challenged with various substances including foods, additives, colorings, chemicals, medicinal herbs, functional foods, molds and pharmaceutical compounds. The patient's unique set of responses help to identify substances that may trigger potentially harmful immune system reactions. The Alcat Test objectively classifies a patient's response to each test substance as reactive, borderline or non-reactive. Based on these classifications, a customized elimination/rotation diet may be designed to effectively eliminate the specific triggers of chronic immune system activation. By reducing this ongoing burden—and in particular, by reversing the sustained and destructive inflammation it produces—normal body functions and immune system balance can be improved.

Go to drcolbert.com to order the Alcat Test.

Appendix E

SUPPLEMENTS

Depending on your health and your sickness, I may suggest one or more supplements to help speed you along the trail toward health. All supplements are recommendations. To review the supplements, go to www.drcolbert.com now. You can order at any time.

Divine Health Nutritional Products
shop.drcolbert.com
(407) 732-6952

1. Green Supremefood: A whole food nutritional powder with fermented grasses and vegetables
2. Red Supremefood: A whole food nutritional powder with anti-aging fruits
3. Fermented Plant Protein
4. Enhanced Multivitamin

Appendix F

GLUTEN IS EVERYWHERE

According to the Celiac Disease Foundation (celiac.org), there are many sources of gluten. The following grains and their derivatives are sources of gluten:

- Wheat: varieties and derivatives of wheat such as: wheatberries, durum, emmer, semolina, spelt, farina, faro, graham, KAMUT° khorasan wheat, einkorn wheat
- Rye
- Barley
- Triticale
- Malt in various forms including: malted barley flour, malted milk or milk shakes, malt extract, malt syrup, malt flavoring, malt vinegar
- Brewer's Yeast
- Wheat starch that has not been processed to remove the presence of gluten to below 20ppm and adhere to the FDA Labeling Law

There are many food items that may contain these sources of gluten, often in hidden or unexpected ways. Always read the labels of any food products you are buying if gluten-free is not specified on the label. Products labeled wheat-free are not necessarily gluten-free. They may still contain spelt (a form of wheat), rye, or barley-based ingredients that are not gluten-free (GF). To confirm if something is gluten-free, be sure to refer to the product's ingredient list.

According to the FDA, if a food contains wheat starch, it may only be labeled gluten-free if that product has been processed to remove gluten, and tests to below 20 parts per million of gluten. With the enactment of this law on August 5, 2014, individuals with celiac disease or gluten intolerance can be assured that a food containing wheat starch and labeled gluten-free contains no more than 20ppm of gluten. If a product labeled gluten-free contains wheat starch in the ingredient list, it must be followed by an asterisk explaining that the wheat has been processed sufficiently to adhere to the FDA requirements for gluten-free labeling.

Common foods that contain gluten:
- Pastas: raviolis, dumplings, couscous, and gnocchi
- Noodles: ramen, udon, soba (those made with only a percentage of buckwheat flour), chow mein, and egg noodles (note: rice noodles and mung bean noodles are gluten free)
- Breads and pastries: croissants, pita, naan, bagels, flatbreads, corn bread, potato bread, muffins, donuts, rolls
- Crackers: pretzels, Goldfish crackers, graham crackers
- Baked goods: cakes, cookies, piecrusts, brownies
- Cereal and granola: corn flakes and rice puffs often contain malt extract/flavoring, granola often made with regular oats not gluten-free oats
- Breakfast foods: pancakes, waffles, French toast, crepes, biscuits
- Breading and coating mixes: panko bread crumbs
- Croutons: stuffings, dressings

- Sauces and gravies (many use wheat flour as a thickener): traditional soy sauce, cream sauces made with a roux
- Flour tortillas
- Beer (unless explicitly gluten-free) and any malt beverages
- Brewer's yeast
- Anything else that uses "wheat flour" as an ingredient

NEXT STEPS

THE TIME TO TAKE ACTION is always now. When it comes to your health and well-being, there is no better time than the present.

I read years ago of a church in Europe that needed a new roof. The massive church had originally been built with huge beams of wood that were both long as well as straight. Without the proper support, the roof's instability could lead to the loss of the church as well as loss of life.

All the old drawings of the building were brought out and studied. On one of the drawings they found a note. It explained how the roof required certain trees for the wood beams, which they already knew, but there was more. The note also contained directions to a field where, more than a century earlier, someone had planted rows of these specific trees that grew tall and straight. They were mature and perfect, ready to be put to use.

Who thinks that way? We may plan ahead a few years, but who thinks 100 years in advance?

I'm challenged *today* to think of my *tomorrows* not just for me, but for my wife, children, grandchildren, and the countless patients I am privileged to serve worldwide.

Though your body naturally craves the very foods that promote disease, you don't have to obey. *You get to choose!*

Though you may have genetics to thank for the predisposition to a disease, they are not the final word. *You get to choose!*

Though it may be tough work to get your health back, it is truly worth it. *You get to choose!*

You have the final word. Each time you make a food choice, it's either a choice that leads to life or one that that leads to death.

Link your passion for living in with your plans for good health and you are on your way to an incredible future!

Let food be your medicine and medicine be your food. Good advice for today . . . and tomorrow.

CONTACTING DR. COLBERT

To contact Dr. Colbert's office, you can do so via:

Internet: www.drcolbert.com
Phone: 407-331-7007
Fax: 407-331-5777
Email: info@drcolbert.com
Facebook: facebook.com/DonColbertMD
Twitter: @DonColbert

NOTES

1. http://www.fda.gov/ForConsumers/ConsumerUpdates/ucm372915.htm
2. http://www.ub.edu/web/ub/en/menu_eines/noticies/2013/02/070.html
3. William Davis, *Wheat Belly* (New York, NY: Rodale, 2011).
4. Ibid.
5. David Perlmutter, *Grain Brain* (New York, NY: Little, Brown and Company, 2013).
6. https://www.organicconsumers.org/news/
   spilling-beans-unintended-gmo-health-risks
7. http://www.centerforfoodsafety.org/issues/311/ge-foods/ge-food-and
   -your-health
8. http://bamboocorefitness.com/not-so-sweet-the-average-american
   -consumes-150-170-pounds-of-sugar-each-year/
9. Daniela Jakubowicz, Maayan Barnea, Julio Wainstein, Oren Froy. "High caloric intake at breakfast vs. dinner differentially influences weight loss of overweight and obese women," Obesity, 2013; DOI: 10.1002/oby.20460.
10. http://www.timesofisrael.com/want-to-lose-weight-make-breakfast-your
    -big-meal-and-have-dessert-with-it/
11. http://www.cdc.gov/heartdisease/facts.htm
12. http://www.forbes.com/sites/leahbinder/2013/09/23/
    stunning-news-on-preventable-deaths-in-hospitals/
13. http://www.healthline.com/health/rheumatoid-arthritis-complications
    #ComplicationsofRheumatoidArthritis1
14. https://www.aaemonline.org/gmo.php
15. http://www.huffingtonpost.com/margie-kelly/genetically-modified-food
    _b_2039455.html
16. Thomas N. Seyfried, *Cancer as a Metabolic Disease: On the Origin, Management, and Prevention of Cancer* (Hoboken, NJ: Wiley, 2012).
17. http://www.alz.org/facts/
18. http://www.mayoclinic.org/diseases-conditions/dementia/basics/prevention
    /con-20034399
19. *AGING*, vol 6, no 9, pp 707–717, The Reversals of Cognitive Decline: A Novel Therapeutic Program by Dale E. Bredesen and Mary S. Easton Center for Alzheimer's Disease Research, Department of Neurology, University of California, Los Angeles, CA 90095 and Buck Institute for Research on Aging, Novato, CA 94945.
20. http://www.fda.gov/Food/IngredientsPackagingLabeling/
    FoodAdditivesIngredients/ucm328728.htm

21. https://food-nutrition.knoji.com/the-facts-about-msg-and-your-health/
22. http://www.healthline.com/health/adhd/facts-statistics-infographic#1
23. http://www.adaa.org/about-adaa/press-room/facts-statistics
24. http://www.adaa.org/about-adaa/press-room/facts-statistics
25. http://www.nimh.nih.gov/health/statistics/prevalence/any-anxiety-disorder-among-adults.shtml
26. http://www.adaa.org/about-adaa/press-room/facts-statistics
27. RC Kessler, WT Chiu, O Demler, EE Walters, "Prevalence, severity, and comorbidity of 12-month DSM-IV disorders in the National Comorbidity Survey Replication," *Arch Gen Psychiatry* 2005;62:617–627; also see http://www.ncbi.nlm.nih.gov/pubmed/15939839
28. CJL Murray, AD Lopez, *The Global Burden of Disease: A Comprehensive Assessment of Mortality and Disability from Diseases, Injuries and Risk Factors in 1990 and Projected to 2020* (Geneva, Switzerland; World Health Organization, 1996).
29. DP Chapman, GS Perry, TW Strine, "The vital link between chronic disease and depressive disorders," *Prev Chronic Dis* 2005;2(1):A14.
30. Brian Mast, *Know Love, Live Loved* (Nashville, TN: Book Ripple, 2015).

ABOUT THE AUTHOR

DON COLBERT, MD graduated from ORU Medical School in 1984. He then moved to Central Florida, where he did his internship and residency at Florida Hospital. For over twenty-five years, Dr. Colbert has practiced medicine in Central Florida. He has been board certified in family practice for over twenty-five years and specializes in anti-aging medicine. Dr. Colbert is also a *New York Times* best-selling author who has written more than forty books.

Dr. Colbert has ministered health and healing to thousands. He is a frequent guest with John Hagee, Joyce Meyer, Kenneth Copeland, James Robison, Jim Bakker, and other leaders in the body of Christ. Dr. Colbert has also been featured on *The Dr. Oz Show*, Fox News, ABC World News, BBC and in *Readers Digest*, *News Week*, *Prevention* magazine, and many others.

Dr. Colbert offers seminars and talks on a variety of topics including "How to Improve Your Health," "The Effects of Stress and How to Overcome It," "Deadly Emotions," and "The 7 Pillars of Health." Through his research and walk with God, Dr.Colbert has been given a unique insight that has helped thousands improve their lives.

IF YOU ENJOYED THIS BOOK, WILL YOU CONSIDER SHARING THE MESSAGE WITH OTHERS?

Mention the book in a blog post or through Facebook, Twitter, Pinterest, or upload a picture through Instagram.

Recommend this book to those in your small group, book club, workplace, and classes.

Head over to facebook.com/DonColbertMD, "LIKE" the page, and post a comment as to what you enjoyed the most.

Tweet "I recommend reading #LetFoodBeYourMedicine by @DonColbert // @worthypub"

Pick up a copy for someone you know who would be challenged and encouraged by this message.

Write a book review online.

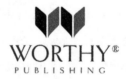

Visit us at worthypublishing.com

twitter.com/worthypub

worthypub.tumblr.com

facebook.com/worthypublishing

pinterest.com/worthypub

instagram.com/worthypub

youtube.com/worthypublishing